Yarn Manufacture

Laboratory Manual-cum-Application Handbook

Volume I

The Authors

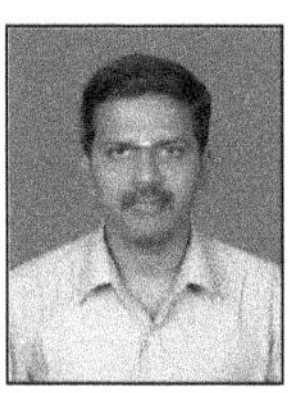

Dr. T. Karthik is presently working as an Assistant Professor (Senior Grade) in the Department of Textile Technology, PSG College of Technology Peelamedu, Coimbatore. He has 5 years teaching, 5 years industrial and 5 years experience of handling various spinning subjects.

He has contributed more than 40 articles in International and National Journals of repute. He has published two books and contributed one book chapter. He is the member in Professional bodies such as TAI and MIE.

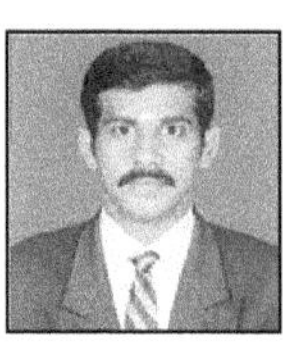

Dr. J.C. Sakthivel is presently working as an Assistant Professor in the Department of Textile Technology, P.S.G. College of Technology, Peelamedu, Coimbatore. He has 12 years of teaching experience. He is actively engaged in handling various subject related to yarn manufacturing, technical textiles and Non wovens.

Dr. Sakthivel has published more than 30 articles in journals of repute. He is the member of professional bodies such as TAI, ISTE and AMIE.

Yarn Manufacture

Laboratory Manual-cum-Application Handbook

Volume I

Authors

Dr. T. Karthik

Dr. J.C. Sakthivel

2016

Daya Publishing House®

A Division of

Astral International Pvt. Ltd.

New Delhi – 110 002

Cataloging in Publication Data--DK
Courtesy: D.K. Agencies (P) Ltd. <docinfo@dkagencies.com>

Karthik, T., author.
Yarn manufacture I : laboratory record-cum-application handbook / authors, Dr. T. Karthik, Dr. J.C. Sakthivel.
pages cm
Includes bibliographical references.
ISBN: 978-93-5130-957-4 (Vol. 1)
ISBN 978-93-5130-924-6 (International Edition)
1. Yarn--Handbooks, manuals, etc. 2. Textile industry--Handbooks, manuals, etc. I. Sakthivel, J. C., author. II. Title.
TS1451.K37 2016 DDC 677.078 23

Published by : **Daya Publishing House®**
A Division of
Astral International Pvt. Ltd.
– ISO 9001:2008 Certified Company –
4760-61/23, Ansari Road, Darya Ganj
New Delhi-110 002
Ph. 011-43549197, 23278134
E-mail: info@astralint.com
Website: www.astralint.com

Laser Typesetting : **Classic Computer Services**, Delhi - 110 035

Printed at : **Replika Press Pvt. Ltd.**

Acknowledgement

We would like to thank the Management and the Principal, PSG College of Technology for providing us the excellent facilities and environment for writing the book. We would like to express our sincere gratitude to Dr.G.Thilagavathi, Professor and Head, Department of Textile Technology, PSG College of Technology for the constant motivation. We would also like to express our sincere gratitude to spinning machinery manufacturers Lakshmi Machine Works, Rieter India Pvt Ltd and Trutzschler for giving us permission to utilize their machinery photographs in the book. Finally, we are thankful to those who have inspired and helped me directly or indirectly in writing this book.

Dr. T. Karthik

Dr. J.C. Sakthivel

Preface

Globally the textile industry is one of the oldest representing fourth largest manufacturing industry with yarn manufacturing as the most valuable component as it is the first process in the supply chain and forming a build block for fabrics. Today textile industry is facing higher competition in the globalized market than ever before. Hence spinning and spinning preparatory is the key process and has vital importance because fabric properties and weaving performance are dependent on yarn quality.

Keeping this in mind, **Yarn Manufacture – I, Laboratory Record-cum-Application Handbook book** outlines the basic principle of operation of fibre preparation machines such as Blow room, Carding and spinning preparation namely, Draw frame. This book is divided into twelve experiments in fibre and spinning preparation, each discusses certain elements in the machine. This book is primarily a text book intended for Textile Technology students in universities and colleges, researchers, industrialists and academicians.

Experiment 1 to 5 presents the various experiments related to Blow room process such as determination of speeds, surface speeds, openness values, blending homogeneity etc. Experiments 6 to 9 discusses experiments related to Carding machines such as draft and draft constant calculations, wire clothing, transfer co-efficient theory etc. Finally, the experiments 10 to 12 provides experiments related to Draw frame such as draft and doubling concepts, roller setting recommendations etc.

The reader is also provided with useful formulas and conversion factors for better understanding.

Dr. T. Karthik

Dr. J.C. Sakthivel

Contents

Spinning Useful Formula

Classification of Cotton

Length [Inch]	$^{13}/_{16}$" to $^{5}/_{16}$"	Short staple
	$^{31}/_{32}$" to $1^{1}/_{8}$"	Medium staple
	$1^{5}/_{32}$" to $1\ ^{1}/_{4}$"	Medium to long staple
	$1^{9}/_{32}$" to $1^{3}/_{8}$"	Long staple
	$1^{13}/_{32}$" to $1^{3}/_{4}$"	Extra long staple
Fineness	Below 3.0	Very fine
[Microgram/inch or	3.0–3.9	Fine
µg/in or Micronaire	4.0–4.9	Average
	5.0–5.9	Rather coarse
	6.0 and higher	Coarse
Breaking Strength	93 and higher	Excellent
[Pressley 1000 lbs/inch^2]	87–92	Very strong
	81–86	Strong
	75–80	Average
	70–74	Passable
	Below 70	Weak

Maturity	82% and higher	Mature
[% Causticaire]	76%–81%	Medium-mature
	70%–75%	Immature
	Below 70%	Very immature
Uster Statistics	5%–10%	Very good
	10%–25%	Good
	25%–50%	Average
	50%–75%	Below average
	75%–95%	Much below average
Shirley-Analyzer	<1.2% Trash	Very clean
[Rieter Standard]	1.21%–2.0%	Clean
	2.01%–4.0%	Average
	4.01%–7.0%	Dirty
	7.01% and more	Very dirty

Spinning Limits

Spinning Limit	*Number of Fibres Ø* $= \frac{\text{tex Yarn}}{\text{tex Fibre}}$
Long staple Material (Wool and Blends)	< 40 Fibres
Staple fibre 3.3dtex / 50-60-80mm	Ø 55–70 Fibres
Staple fibre 1.3-1.7dtex / 38-40mm	Ø 70–80 Fibres
Cotton – Ring yarn, Cotton – Rotor yarn	Ø 120–150 Fibres

Yarn Break Standards

Yarn breaks/100 Spd/h or R/h — *Yarn break/100 h* $= \frac{\text{Yarn break} \times 1000}{\text{Run-time/h} \times \text{No. Spd/h}}$

CO Combed Ring Yarn	*CO Carded Ring Yarn*	*Long Staple 100%*	*Rotor Yarn*	*Rating*
12	14	38	20	Good
23	28	75	30	Average
48	58	150	55	Poor

Quality Values

A%	Mean deviation of the count from the set value as determined with reference to a defined duration (almost shift)
U%	Count variation = out-of-date
	CV% =1.25•U%
CV%	Coefficient of variation of evenness
	$CV = S/\overline{X}$
	s = Standard deviation, $\overline{X}$ = Mean value
CVL x m	Coefficient of variation of count for the set cut length x
	x = 1m, 3m, 10m, 100m, or yards
Sliver count spectrogram	Graphic depiction of periodically occurring unevenness (Peak) = Poisson distribution
	Range or wavelength, which the data system can measure: a few cm to several 100m

Basic Conversion Charts

	Name of the Unit	*Symbol*	*Metric unit*
Length unit	1 inch	in	2.54 cm
	1 foot (=12 in)	ft	0.3048 m
	1 yard (=3ft)	yd	0.9144 m
	1 mile		1609.344 m
Area units	1 square inch	sq in	6.4516 cm^2
	1 square foot	sq ft	929.030 cm^2
	1 square yard	sq yd	0.836127 m^2
Mass units	1 grain	gr	0.064799 g
	1 ounce	oz	28.3495 g
	1 pound (=10 oz)	lb	0.453592 kg
Force units	1 ounce-force	ozf	0.278014 N
	1 pound-force (=16 ozf)	lbf	4.44822 N
Pressure units	1 pound-force per square inch	lbf/in^2	6894.76 N/m^2
	1 pound-force per square foot	lbf/ft^2	47.8803 N/m^2
Tenacity	1 kilogram-force. Ne	1 kgf.Ne_c	0.579 cN/tex
	1 gram-force per denier	1 gf/den	8.838 cN/tex

Temperature	*1° Fahrenheit*	°F	$\frac{°F-32}{1.8}$ *1.8*
	1° Celsius	°C	*1.8x °C + 32[°F]*

°F	50	60	65	70	75	80	85	90	100
°C	10	16	18	21	24	27	29	32	38

Sliver Weight from Metric to Imperial Units

g/m	20	30	40	50	55	60	65	70	75	80	85	90	100
gr/yd	282	423	564	706	776	847	917	988	1058	1129	1199	1270	1411

Yarn Count System

The weight system	$tex = \frac{m}{l}$ (g/km) dtex for fibres tex for yarn ktex for slivers	The unit **tex** reveals how many Grams per 1000 m, a product weighs.
The length system	$Nm = \frac{1}{m}$ (m/g, mm/mg, km/kg)	*i.e.* **Nm 10** defines, that 10 m Material weigh 1 Gram.
	$Ne = \frac{\text{Hank (840 yd)}}{\text{Pound (lb)}}$	*i.e.* **Nec 60** defines, that 60 Hank (840 yd) weigh 1 Pound (lb)
Conversion	$Nm = \frac{1000}{tex}$ $Ne = \frac{590.541}{tex}$ Ne = 0.590541 x Nm, Nm = 1.69336 x Ne dtex = μg/in x 0.394 (μg/in = micronaire)	

Twist	*Twist Multiplier*
With N_e, $T/in = \alpha e \times \sqrt{Ne}$	With N_e, $\alpha_e = \frac{T/in}{\sqrt{Ne}}$
With N_m, $T/m = \alpha m \times \sqrt{Nm}$	
With tex, $T/m = \alpha tex/\sqrt{tex}$	With N_m, $\alpha_m = \frac{T/m}{\sqrt{Nm}}$
$T/m = T/in \times 39.4$; $T/in = T/m \times 0.0254$	
Weft twist = Warp x 0.9	With tex, $\alpha_{tex} = T/m \times \sqrt{tex}$
Knit twist = Warp x 0.8	

from to	α_{tex}	α_m	α_e
α_{tex}	—	$31.6 \times \alpha_m$	$957 \times \alpha_e$
α_m	α_{tex} 31.6	—	$30.3 \times \alpha_e$
α_e	α_{tex} 957	α_m30.3	—

Formulas

1. Production in kgs/shift =

$$\frac{\text{Delivery speed (in/min)} \times 60 \times 8 \times \text{machine efficiency \%}}{36 \times 840 \times 2.204 \times \text{Count (Ne)} \times 100}$$

2. $$\text{Draft} = \frac{\text{Surface speed of delivery roller in inch/min}}{\text{Surface speed of feed roller inch/min}}$$

3. In the case of 3/3 drafting system

   a) $$\text{Break Draft (D1)} = \frac{\text{Surface speed of middle roller}}{\text{Surface speed of back roller}}$$

   b) $$\text{Main Draft (D2)} = \frac{\text{Surface speed of front roller}}{\text{Surface speed of middle roller}}$$

   c) $$\text{Total Draft (D3)} = \frac{\text{Surface speed of front roller}}{\text{Surface speed of back roller}}$$

   $$= D1 \times D2$$

$$\text{Twist (TPI)} = \frac{\text{Spindle speed (in rpm)}}{\text{Delivery speed (incher/min)}}$$

$$= \text{Twist Multiplier} \times \sqrt{\text{count}}$$

Count Conversion Chart

	tex	dtex	den	gr/yd	micron	Nm	Ne	NeK	NeW
tex	1	dtex X 0.1	den X 0.111	(gr/yd) X 70.86	micron/25.4	1,000/Nm	590.5/NeC	885.5/NeW	1,937.7/NeW
dtex	tex X 10	1	den X 1.11	(gr/yd) X 708.6	micron/2.54	10,000/Nm	5,905.4/NeC	8,858/NeW	19,377/NeW
den	tex X 9	dtex X 0.9	1	(gr/yd) X 637.7	micron/2.82	9,000/Nm	5,314.9/NeC	7,972.3/NeK	17,439/NeW
gr/yd	tex/70.86	tex/708.6	den/637.7	1	micron/1801.4	14.1/Nm	8.33/NeC	12.5/NeK	27.34/NeW
micron	tex X 25.4	dtex X 2.54	den X 2.82	gr/yd X 1801.4	1	25,400/ Nm	15,000/NeC	22,500/NeK	49,218/NeW
Nm	1000/tex	10,000/dtex	9,000/den	14.1/(gr/yd)	25,400/micron	1	NeC X 1.693	NeK / 1.5	NeW X0.516
Ne	590.5/tex	5905.4/dtex	5314.9/den	8.33/(gr/yd)	15,000/micron	Nm/1.693	1	NeK/1.5	NeW/3.28
NeK	882.8/tex	8858/dtex	7972.3/den	12.5/(gr/yd)	22,500/micron	Nm/1.13	NeC X 1.5	1	NeW/2.187
NeW	1,937.7/tex	19,377/dtex	17,439/den	27.34/(gr/yd)	49,218/micron	Nm/0.516	NeC X 3.28	NeK X 2.187	1

- ✓ dtex = Decitex
- ✓ den = Denier
- ✓ Micron = micron per inch (Micronaire type instrument)
- ✓ Nm = Number
- ✓ Metric Count System NeC = Number English Cotton Count System
- ✓ NeK = Number English Worsted Count System
- ✓ NeW = Number English Woollen Count System

Simplified Formulas

1. Ring frame production/spindle/8 hrs (g) =

$$\frac{7.2 \times \text{spindle speed (rpm)} \times \text{m/c eff (\%)}}{\text{Count} \times \text{TPI} \times 100}$$

2. Speed frame production/spindle/8 hrs (kgs) =

$$\frac{7.2 \times \text{spindle speed (rpm)} \times \text{m/c eff (\%)}}{\text{Count} \times \text{TPI} \times 100000}$$

3. Drawframe production/delivery/8 hrs (kgs) =

$$\frac{0.2835 \times \text{delivery speed (mpm)} \times \text{m/c eff (\%)}}{\text{Sliver hank} \times 100}$$

4. Card production/delivery/8 hrs =

$$\frac{0.2835 \times \text{delivery speed (mpm)} \times \text{m/c efficiency (\%)}}{\text{Sliver hank} \times 100}$$

5. Production/scutcher/8 hrs (kg) =

$$\frac{0.2835 \times \text{delivery speed (mpm)} \times \text{m/c eff (\%)}}{\text{Lap hank} \times 100}$$

CYCLE OF CARDED COTTON

stage	machine	entry material	delivery material	package form
Opening and cleaning	bale plucker, opener, blender	raw cotton	lap	---
Carding	card	lap	card sliver	can
1st drawing	drawframe	card sliver	drawn sliver	sliver can
2nd drawing	drawframe	drawn sliver	drawn sliver	roving can
Roving	roving frame	drawn sliver	roving	roving bobbin
Spinning	ring spinning frame	roving	ring-spun yarn	bobbin / spool / cheese
Post-spinning processes	winding, doubling, singeing, reeling, twisting, winding-off machines	yarn	yarn	various (skein, bobbin, package)

The *conventional process of cotton spinning* can be considered broken down into four processing stages:

a) *Opening, blending and cleaning* the fibre, carried out in order to permit the tufts to recovery their natural softness, which is lessened when the cotton is pressed into bales; blending the fibre must be as accurate as possible; a system of staves, batten reels and grids contribute to eliminating most of the natural impurities contained in cotton tufts; then puckers, openers and blenders are used;

b) *Disentangling*, achieved by beating and carding, needed for increasing the relative parallelization of the fibres, obtains a clean product free from fibres that are too short;

c) *Doubling*, consists in drawing near and processing similar products (card and drawn sliver) from various machines, in order to improve the homogenous nature of semi-processed goods and consequentially the yarn, permitting any eventual irregular sections to be identified and homogenized;

d) *Preparation for spinning and spinning*, this is actually the transformation of the semi-processed product to yarn with the desired properties (count, twist) and it is obtained using roving frames, followed by ring spinning frame;

e) *Complementary processing*, supplementary operations necessary only for obtaining a certain packaging or a particular look for the final product; these operations are: doubling, twisting, winding, singeing, reeling and winding-off.

COMBED COTTON SPINNING

stage	machine	entry material	delivery material	package form
Opening and cleaning	bale plucker, opener, blender	raw cotton	lap	---
Carding	card	lap	card sliver	drawn lap can
Pre-comber drawing	drawframe / lap drawing frame	card sliver	drawn lap	drawn lap can
Combing	combing machine	drawn lap	comb sliver	comb sliver can
Post-comber drawing	drawframe	comb sliver	drawn sliver	roving can
Roving	roving frame	drawn sliver	roving	roving bobbin
Spinning	ring spinning frame	roving	Ring-spun yarn	bobbin / spool / cheese
Post-spinning processes	Winding, doubling, singeing, reeling, twisting, winding-off machines	yarn	yarn	various (skein, bobbin, package)

ROTOR COTTON SPINNING

stage	machine	entry material	delivery material	Package form
Opening and cleaning	bale plucker, opener, blender	raw cotton	lap	---
Carding	card	lap	card sliver	can
Drawing	drawframe	card sliver	drawn sliver	drawframe can
Spinning	open-end spinning frame	drawn sliver	(O-E) yarn	package

1

Working Mechanism of Mixing Bale Opener and Automatic Bale Opener

1. AIM

- ☆ To draw the gearing diagram of the machine.
- ☆ To observe the design features and important functional elements of the machine / mechanism.
- ☆ To calculate the speed of various elements and production of the machine.
- ☆ To study the working of Automatic Bale Opener.

2. FORMULA

Refer spinning useful formula relevant to your experiment

3. DESCRIPTION

The blowroom should function to:

- ☆ mix and open the fibres,
- ☆ remove an optimal amount of trash
- ☆ minimize nep formation
- ☆ minimize fibre damage.
- ☆ minimize the loss of good fibre in the waste.

A goal of the blowroom is to:

- ☆ remove 70 to 75% of the trash in the bales
- ☆ not increase the nep level by more than 100%
- ☆ not increase the short fibre content (SFC)
- ☆ not reduce the staple length of the fibre.

Functions of the Blowroom

Opening

The Need for Opening

- ☆ To clean, mix and blend fibres they have to be brought into the smallest aggregate form. The baled material has to be re-opened and fed in small tufts as part of the overall preparation process. Only well opened material can be effectively cleaned.
- ☆ To enable the fibres to be blended they must be thoroughly opened.
- ☆ To prepare the fibres for the carding and subsequent operations they must be opened to the point where there will be minimal fibre damage.

Observations about Fibre Opening

- ☆ Opening and cleaning machines should constitute a unit, so that the tuft surfaces are cleaned before they are consolidated in the transportation system.
- ☆ Opening must be performed effectively with the least number of machines.
- ☆ More than four opening operations, prior to carding, will usually not improve the fibre quality. Excessive opening increases the number of neps in the cotton.
- ☆ Feeding tufts in "free motion" permits cleaning but no opening.
- ☆ Feeding the material in a firmly held state is used for intensive opening.
- ☆ Pins, spikes and teeth open fibres more effectively than bars or slats.
- ☆ The higher the degree of opening in the blowroom, the cleaner can be the material fed to the card and consequently a cleaner sliver is produced.
- ☆ The material flow rates through each machine in the blowroom should be adjusted to minimize standing time waiting to feed the next machine. The machines should run between 85% and 90% of the time

Cleaning

The Need for Cleaning

The trash and other impurities contained in cotton received by the spinner must be removed as completely as possible to enable an effective spinning operation to be performed at high speeds. The exception to the above statement applies to spinners of novelty yarns and those who spin "low end" very coarse yarns.

Well-cleaned cotton enables the spinner to,

- ✰ Minimize ends down in spinning,
- ✰ Reduce the weak places caused by trash in the yarn,
- ✰ Spin fine yarns,
- ✰ Produce a more uniform yarn and fabric,
- ✰ Obtain a clean yarn and fabric,
- ✰ Improve downstream processing efficiencies.

Factors Influencing Cleaning

- ✰ Normally trash is separated from the cotton by centrifugal force.
- ✰ The material is moved at high speed in a circular motion.
- ✰ The trash tends to sling out from the fibre surface.
- ✰ Grid bars are provided to allow the trash to escape and separate from the fibre that passes over the grid bars.
- ✰ The grid bars are adjustable to vary the angle and open space allowing more, or less trash to be removed.
- ✰ With an increase in the grid bar opening, there is an increase in the amount of good fibre that goes into the waste with the trash.
- ✰ Good fibre in the waste is normally kept to a minimal amount. However, if maximum cleaning is required there will be good fibre in the waste.
- ✰ New tuft surfaces must be created continuously to facilitate cleaning.
- ✰ Larger, heavier particles are relatively easy to remove.
- ✰ Beating devices tend to break large trash particles making them smaller and more difficult to remove. Large trash should be removed at the beginning of the cleaning process. For this reason, cotton removed from the bales should be in small tufts for effective cleaning.
- ✰ Very small trash particles tend to be carried with the cotton in the transport air and it is difficult to obtain separation. Condensers and fibre separators help with the removal of dust sized particles.

MIXING BALE OPENER (MBO)

The constructional details of machine are shown in sectional drawing (Figure 1.1). The cotton passes over the feed belt at the front into the very spacious mixing bin, having a height of 2m. From here the cotton is conveyed by the slightly inclined bottom apron on to the upright lattice which carries it upwards. While the intake of material is controlled by a counter weighted regulating spade. The close fine and staggered arrangement of the spikes of the upright lattice prevents the formation of 'lanes' in the material. The regulating roller also has staggered spikes and is the first unit which opens the cotton, throwing the unopened lumps back into the mixing bin. To prevent the formation of laps and to assist opening, a clearer roller engages its spikes in those of the regulating roller. The bearings of both rollers are carried in a

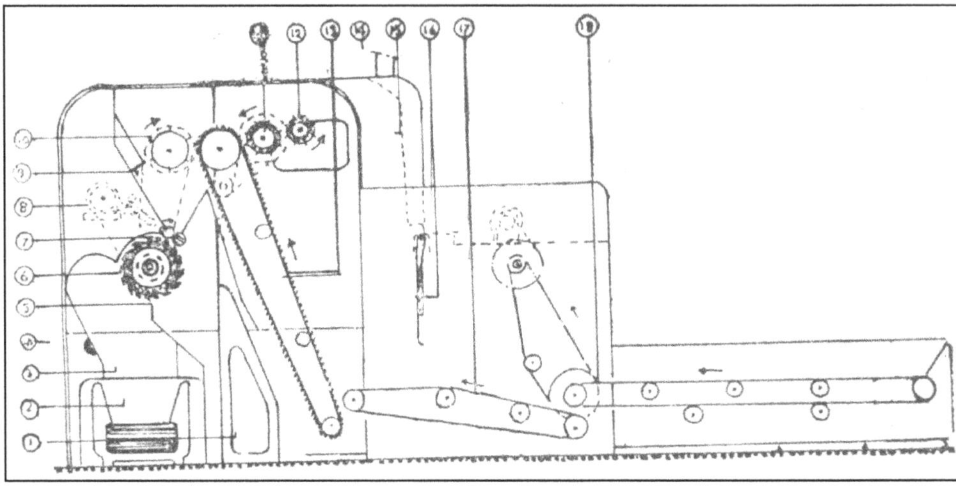

Figure 1.1

1: Waste Space; 2: Conveyor Belt; 3: Outlet; 4: Permanent Magnet; 5: Grid; 6: Opening Cylinder; 7: Pair of Feed Rollers; 8: Two Motors; 9: Trunk; 10: Stripper Roller; 11: Regulating Roller; 12: Clearer Roller; 13: Upright Lattice; 14: Connection for Dust Exhaustion; 16: Perforated sheet; 16: Regulating Spade; 17: Rubber Apron; 18: Feed Belt.

bracket and they can be adjusted sleeplessly in relation to the upright lattice during operation by means of a hand wheel so as to regulate the flow of material in accordance with the production required. Due to the large working space, short length of the roller and lattice spikes and the low operation speed, very thorough but careful loosening is achieved and the longer turning over period for each constituent of the blend ensures more effective mixing.

Opening Cylinder with Adjustable Grid

Already well opened by upright lattice, the cotton flocks are taken off by a stripper roller provided with strips of rubber and thrown into the trunk, which guides them into the pair of feed rollers. Here the cotton is beaten off the spring loaded feed roller by the opening saw toothed cylinder and led the material into outlet over a grid. This beating action divides the material into smallest flocks, at the same time removing a large part of the impurities without damaging the fibres. The setting of the grid can be changed easily and centrally during operation. With correct adjustment optimum results can be quickly obtained for any cotton.

Waste space and dust exhaustion

The large waste space underneath the grid is easily accessible by means of doors on either side, so that removal of the waste is perfectly straight forward. It can be combined with central waste collecting arrangement in case of an automated spinning mill. Dust exhaustion is effected through connection located above the feed or mixing bin, through a perforated sheet which prevents good fibres from being carried along. All mixing bale openers of the same opener line are connected to the one central fan.

Installation of Permanent Magnet

Three or more mixing bale openers, throw the cotton on to a collecting conveyor belt. In the outlet funnel of which permanent magnets are fitted, so that virtually all particles of iron are extracted from the cotton fibres, making a substantial contribution

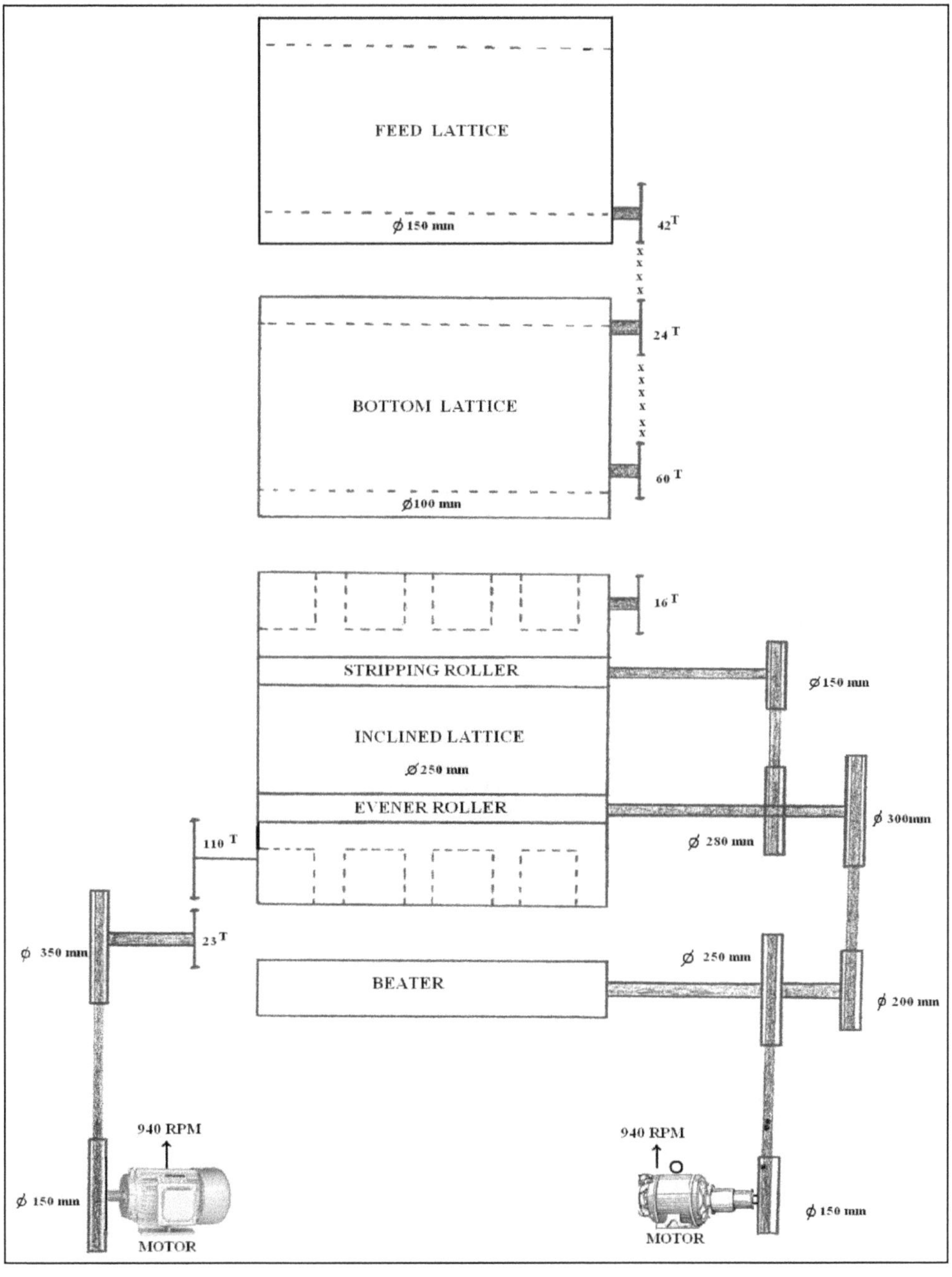

Figure 1.2: Mixing Bale Opener.

towards trouble free operation in the blow room. With smaller opener sequences the cotton falls into an outlet funnel and is taken away pneumatically. In this case permanent magnets are fitted in the outlet of the mixing bale opener.

AUTOMATIC BALE OPENERS

The Rieter UNIfloc enables up to 130 bales arranged per side as four components per blend over a maximum layout length of 50 m to be processed. The machine can process one or two blends simultaneously. The production rate is normally up to 1400 kg/hr.

The feed duct and the two guide rails are secured to the floor. The chassis, which moves back and forth on the guide rails, carries a turret, which is rotatable through 1800 and supports a risible and lower able extracting assembly. The latter has individually replaceable double-tooth discs and changes its direction of rotation on reversal of the direction of movement of the chassis, so that material can be extracted in both directions of travel.

4. PROCEDURE

1. Draw the complete gearing diagram of the machine
2. Show by arrow the flow of motion starting from motor to various parts
3. Mark various change pulleys / gears
4. Note down the diameters of the pulleys number of teeth of the gears and number of rows of spikes on evener roller.
5. Measure the distance between the spikes of the inclined lattice along with their dimensions

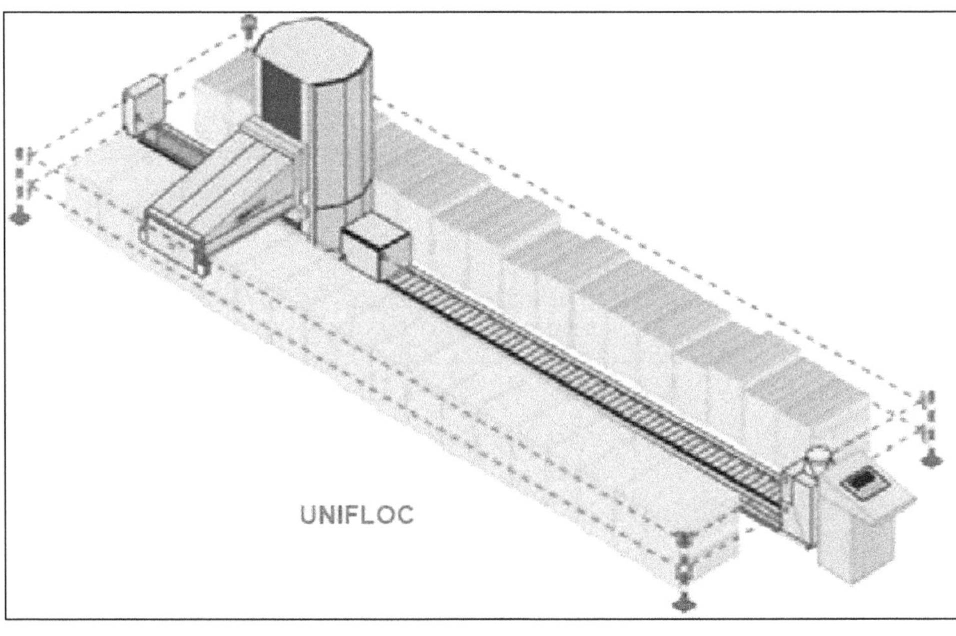

Figure 1.3(a)

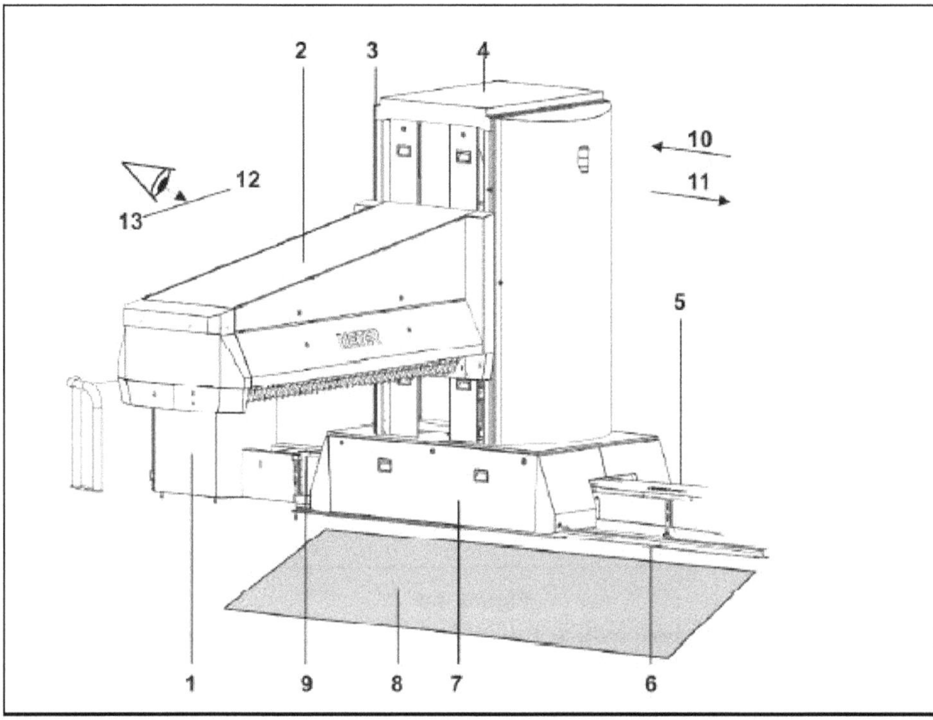

1 Operator panel
2 Take-off unit
3 Electrical control cabinet
4 Rotating tower
5 Tuft chute
6 Rail
7 Drive frame
8 Bale lay-down area
9 Material delivery area
10 Backwards travel direction
11 Backwards travel direction
12 Left side of machine
13 Right side of machine

Figure 1.3(b)

6. Note down the speed and diameter of the motor pulley.
7. List the various setting points.

5. CALCULATIONS

1. Calculate the rotational speeds of evener, doffer stripper rollers and the pulleys driving spiked and bottom lattices. (Speed ratios are inversely proportional to the diameter ratios of the pulleys). Allow 3% belt slippage.
2. Determine spikes / m^2.
3. Determine the number of rows of evener spikes passing per linear meter movement of spiked lattice.

   Let the speed of evener roller = X

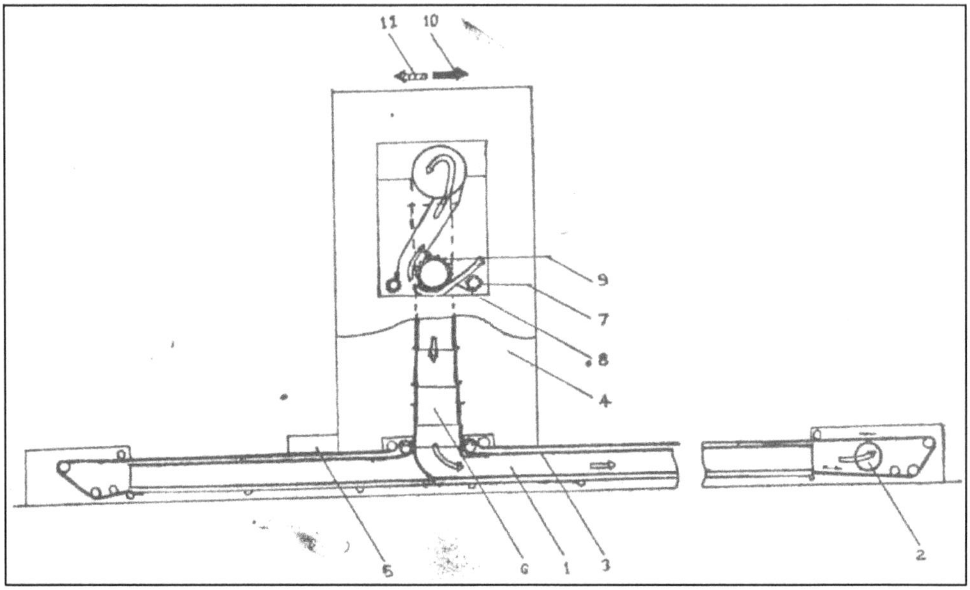

Figure 1.4

1: Sunction duct; 2: Materim exit; 3: Cover belt; 4: Truck with turret; 5: Truck drive; 6: Telescopic tube; 7: Supporting grid; 8: Alternating grid; 9: Toothed disc rollers; 10: Working direction; 11: Return direction.

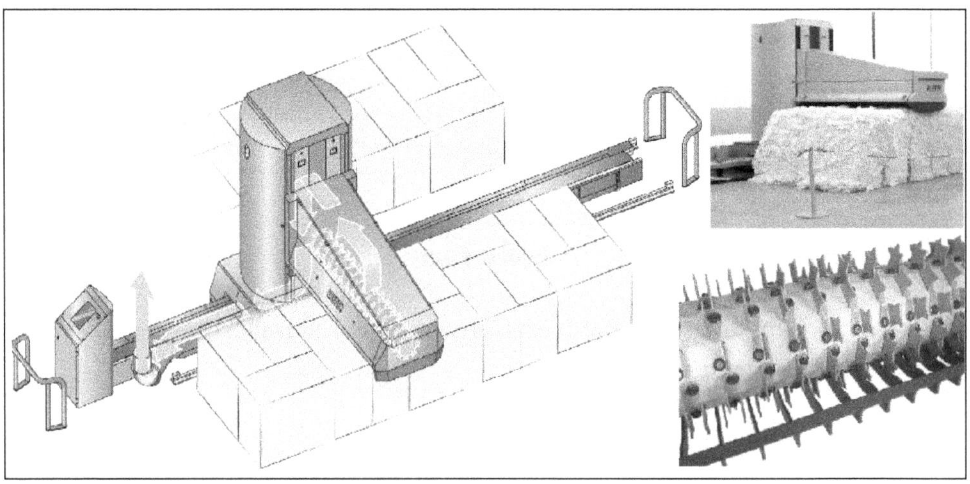

Figure 1.5

No. of rows of spikes on its surface = 4

Surface speed of spiked lattice = V m/min

The above mentioned ration will be 4 X/V

7. RESULTS

Tabulate the results.

	Evener Roller	*Stripper Roller*	*Doffer Roller*	*Bottom Lattice*	*Spiked Lattice*
Rotational speed					
Surface speed					
Spikes/m^2					

2

Working Mechanism of Beaters and Cleaning Machines

1. AIM

- ☆ To draw the motion transmission path from motor to various parts of the machine.
- ☆ To observe the design features and important functional elements of the machine / mechanism
- ☆ To study the working of types of beaters used in blow room line.
- ☆ To calculate the speeds of beater, feed rollers, delivery rollers, fan and cage.

2. FORMULA

Refer spinning useful formula relevant to your experiment

3. DESCRIPTION

PRE-CLEANING MACHINES

1. Mono Cylinder

This is a loose feeding with pin opener. Mono-cylinder cleaner (Figure 2.1) is employed in the blowing room process between the mixing bale opener and auto mixer. Correct connection to the pneumatic conveying system ensures a constant under-pressure in the machine. The advantage of this machine is that the impurities are separated without being crushed and this proves favourable during subsequent operations when the cotton is further processed.

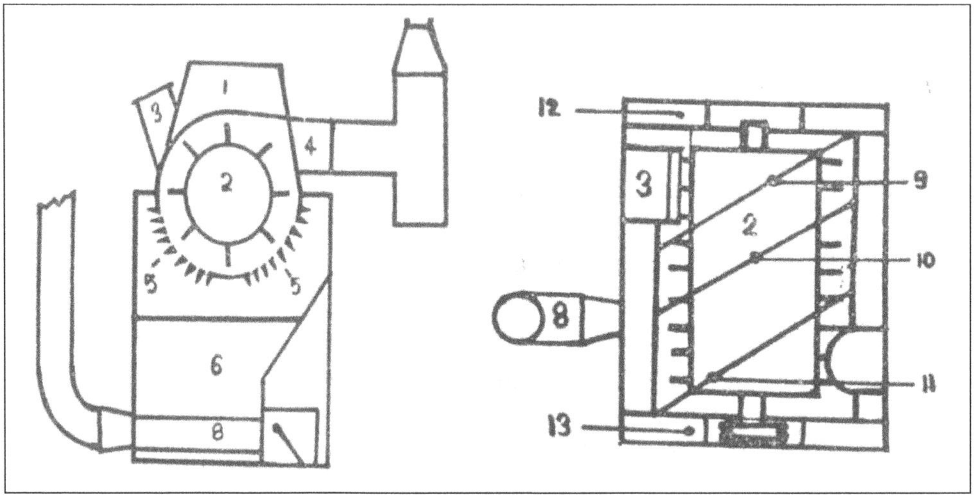

Figure 2.1

1: Hood with guide plates; 2: Pin cylinder; 3: Outlet pipe; 4: Inlet pipe; 5: Adjustable grid; 6: Waste chamber; 7: Engine compartment; 8: Waste remova; 9-11: Guide plates; 12-13: Hinged doors.

The cotton tufts well opened by the bale openers enter the machine at right angles to the cylinder axis. A considerable proportion of the impurities are extracted right at the start by the collision with the pin cylinder and the acceleration in the opposite direction which immediately follows. The pin cylinder then guides the tufts over the grid. Since the tufts are turned over several times as they are flung up, they are brought into contact with the grid on all sides.

This sequence explains the extremely efficient yet gentle cleaning action of mono-cylinder cleaner. Furthermore, the entire cleaning process is repeated three times as the guide plates fitted at an angle to the beater axis into the hood to compel every single tuft to fly round the pin cylinder following a spiral path.

The tangential arrangement of the outlet, branch causes the tufts to emerge along their natural exit path, thereby preventing any addying. The hood with its three guide plates can be opened upwards for cleaning. The cylinder has eight pins around its circumference and six along its length, arranged spirally. The cylinder is fitted with ball bearings at both ends.

Hinged doors opening at the ends permit easy access to the well protected grid adjusting mechanism. The grids are arranged in two separate sections which can be adjusted individually. The grid can be adopted to handle any degree of impurity and opening in the cotton to be processed by means of the levers provided with the scales. The grid can be adjusted regarding spacing (20 to 26 mm) between the grid bars, as well as inclination (0° to 30°)

2. UNIclean/Vario Clean

The UNIclean (Figure 2.2) is an outgrowth of Rieter's experience in removing trash from cotton while it is airborne as the first cleaning point in the blowroom and is consistent with the cleaning philosophy:

- ☆ A minimum number of cleaning positions
- ☆ Maximum working efficiency
- ☆ Optimum fibre preservation
- ☆ High raw material yield

In contrast to conventional pre-cleaners, *i.e.* single-cylinder cleaners or horizontal cleaners, material transport inside the UNIclean takes place mechanically by means of special pins, independently of the conveying air. The raw material is forced over the cleaning grid bars where trash is removed and an integrated de-dusting unit to remove fine particles. The waste is collected inside the machine and is automatically released to the waste suction system.

Since dust and sand cause considerable problems in the spinning operations, the UNIclean has been equipped with an integrated dedusting unit. Dust, sand, some pepper trash and fibre fragments are separated from the cotton by a perforated plate and released to the filter system. Only some 0.5 cubic m/s of dust laden exhaust air has to be removed in the dedusting function.

To control the cleaning action of the UNIclean both the "cleaning intensity" and the "waste rate" have to be programmed into the machine. The cleaning intensity controls both the speed of the drum and a compensatory setting of the grid bars. Increasing the "cleaning intensity" increases the trash removal. The "waste rate" changes the grid angle to remove more or less material. These setting are made on the machine control panel or in the VarioSet program if it is available.

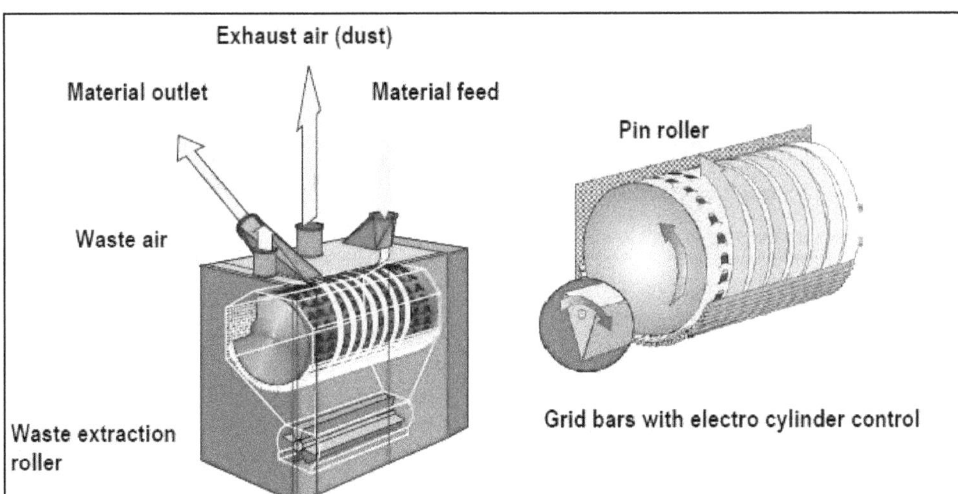

Figure 2.2: UNIclean

Fibre Transportation

The material is blown to the UNIclean, and is circulated seven times inside the machine by the hooks on the drum. The cleaned fibre is sucked from the machine by the transportation fan. Careful adjustment of the airflow is essential to the effective operation of the machine.

Part of the feed transport air is sucked through the perforated plate by the dust waste fan. Fine particles are removed and discharged to the filter system.

The quantity of air required to transport the fibre to the next machine exceeds that amount passing through the machine. To minimize the volume of air passing through the machine, a supplementary air inlet is provided to allow extra air to be sucked into the system as needed.

Cleaning Process

As the fibres enter the machine they are carried in a circular motion by the tines. The fibres are directed by the guide plates to make seven revolutions before leaving the machine. In each revolution the fibres pass the grid bars and the perforated plate. The "Cleaning Intensity" can be adjusted step-less, to changing the rotational speed of the drum. The adjustment can be done while the machine is running. Additionally, the angle of the grid bars is automatically changed in combination with the speed. The "Waste rate" can be varied by changing the grid bar angle with an electrically controlled cylinder. The settings of the cleaning intensity and waste rate can be recalled and used again at a later date.

Cleaning Intensity

Production	*Setting Drum Speed*	
Upto 1200 kg/h	0.0 (low)	480 rpm
	Step-less adjustment to	
	1.0 (high)	960 rpm

Relative Waste Rate

Setting «1» (Low)	*Setting «10» (High):*
Grid closed, lowest waste rate	*Grid open, highest waste rate*
Dark waste composition	*Light-colored waste composition*

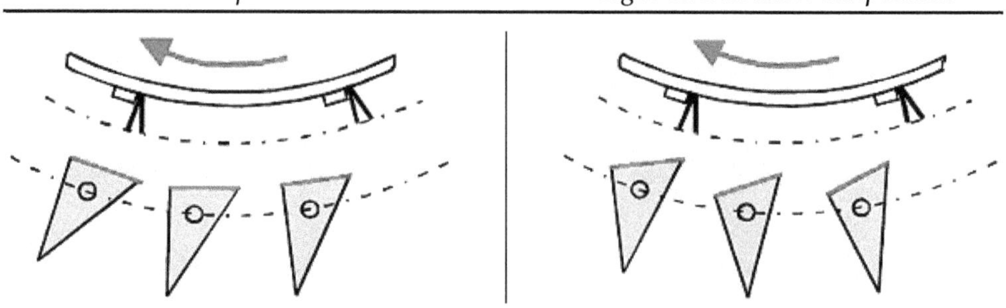

Figure 2.3: Cleaning Characteristic Diagram.

The typical amount of waste to be removed by varying the settings is shown in the following chart. The influence of the cleaning intensity setting increases as the waste rate is increased.

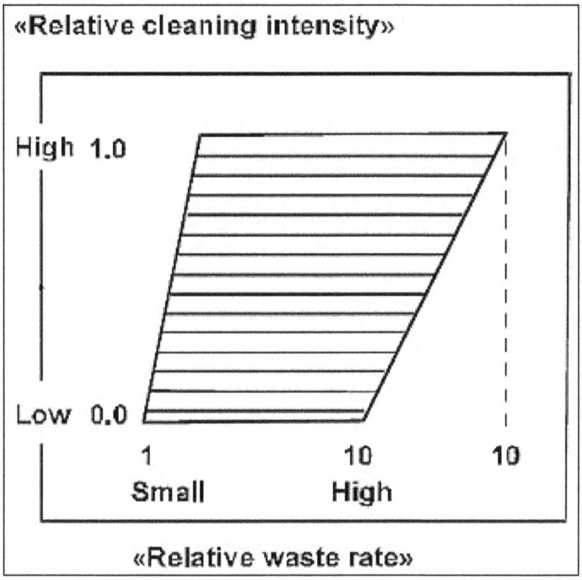

Figure 2.4

As a guideline, the following table gives values of the cleaning intensity and the waste rate according to the trash content of the cotton to be cleaned.

Trash in Cotton	*Applications*	*Cleaning Intensity*	*Waste Rate*
0.5 to 2.0%	Clean cotton fine combed yarns	0.5 to 0.9	0.5 – 0.8%
1.0 to 3.5%	Ring spun carded yarns	0.6 to 0.9	0.8 – 1.5%
1.5 to 4.5%	Rotor yarns Ne 10/1 to 24/1	0.7 to 0.9	1.0 – 2.0%
3.0 to 6.0% and more	Rotor yarns coarse counts	0.2 to 0.7	1.5 – 4.0%

Waste Disposal

The waste is removed periodically through the airlock roller. The interval is determined by the waste transport system. The waste extraction roll incorporates an airlock with seals in waste chamber to prevent excessive good fibre being pulled out with the waste.

Determining the Amount of Waste

To determine the amount of waste extracted, the waste has to be removed by hand, weighed and compared with the production rate to calculate waste%. Follow the instructions on how to isolate the trash chamber from the suction system and manually operate the air lock roller to remove the trash

- ☆ Take at least three (3) tests, each of at least half an hour.
- ☆ (For a provisional test, collect the waste for more than one complete cycle of the UNIfloc.)
- ☆ Record the running time of each test.
- ☆ Calculate the production (kg) during the test time = Carding production rate from the line kg/h x test time in min/60

$$\text{Waste \%} = \frac{\text{Amount of waste removed} \times 100}{\text{Production during test + waste}}$$

Note

The system should be operating with an acceptable stop/go ratio otherwise when the system is optimized the actual waste% will vary from the tested value.

$$\text{Stop/go ratio} = \frac{\text{Running time of the UNIfloc (operating hours counter)}}{\text{Actual time}}$$

FINE-CLEANING MACHINES (Figures 2.5 and 2.6)

The machine consists of the following units

1. Input unit
2. Patented laminar chute
3. Cleaning unit with waste compartment

Input Unit

The fibre is blown into the laminar chute by an integrated fan. The transport air bringing the fibre tufts from the preceding machine compresses the fibre in the chute and escape through the laminar back wall. At the lower end of the laminar feed chute the air enters a perforated drum. The filling of the chute is monitored by 2 photo cells. The air containing dust is passed on to the central filter unit through a duct.

Laminar Chute

The laminar chute is specially designed with T-shaped sections which are self cleaning, further, as there is no leakage of air, the size of the fan motor and the capacity of the filter installation is determined by the energy consumed by the air current conveying the material.

Cleaning Unit

The cleaning unit consists of a spring loaded pair of feed rollers, the knife guide and the cleaning roller. These three units can be optionally adjusted in relation to

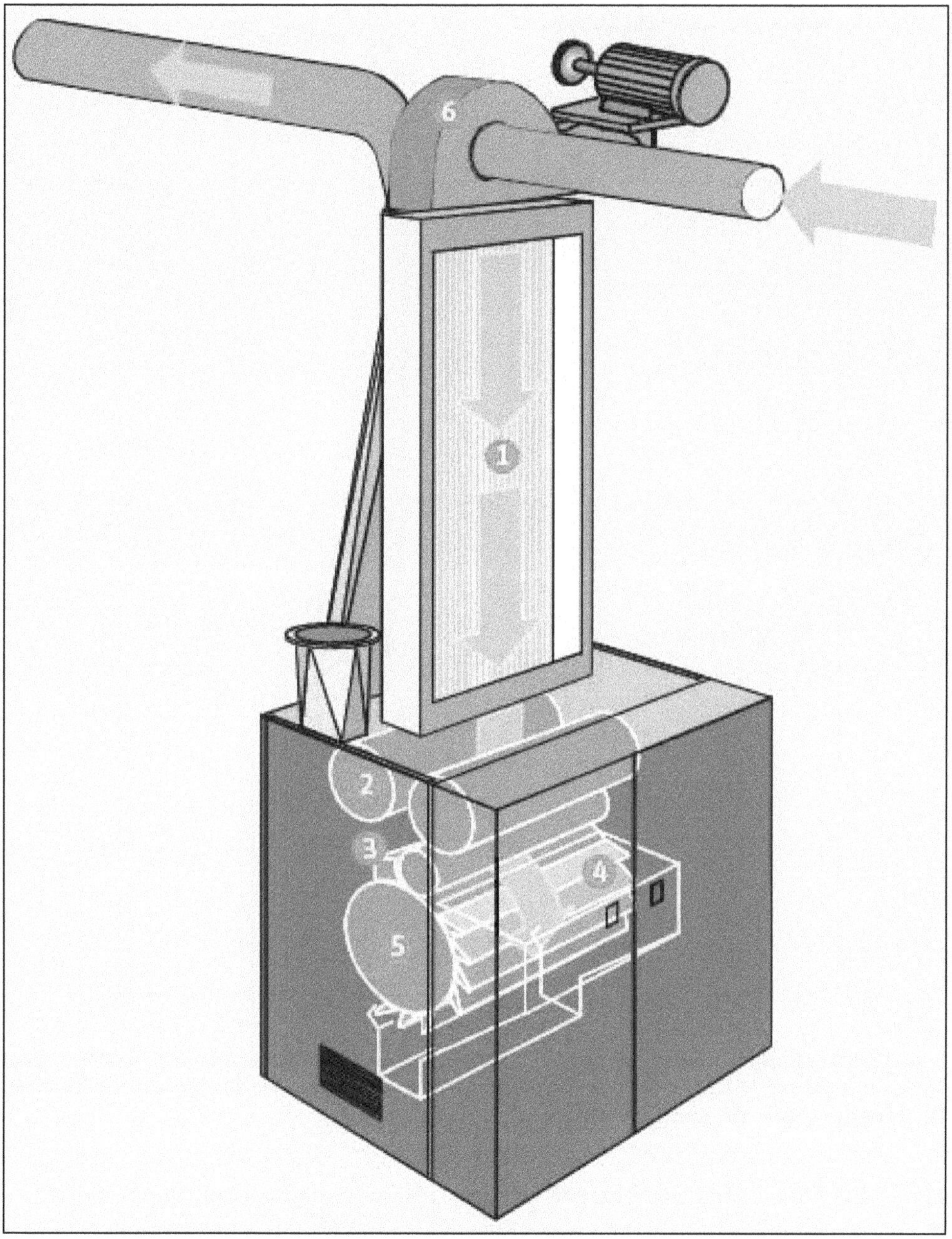

Figure 2.5: Flexi Clean

1: Lamellar chute; 2: Perforated drum; 3: Adjustable feed trough; 4: Adjustable grid; 5: Opening and cleaning cylinder; 6: Fan with divider element.

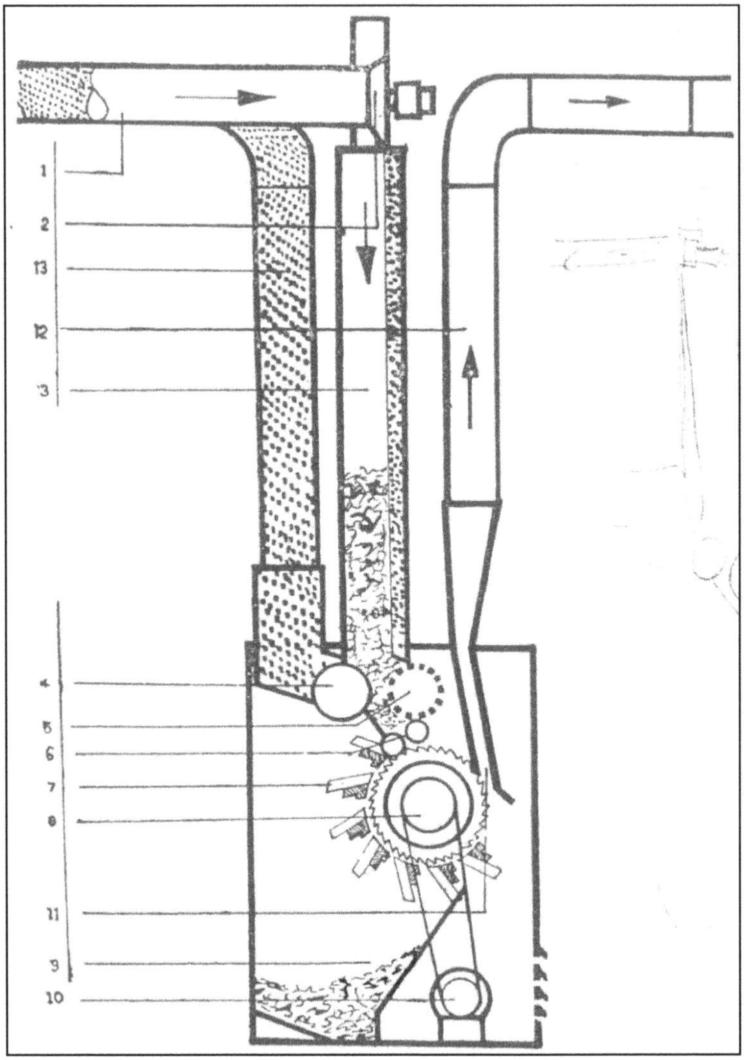

Figure 2.6: : Flexi Clean

1: Material supply; 2: Feeding heed; 3: Laminar trunk; 4: Plain drum; 5: Dust cager; 6: Feed rollers; 7: Knife grid; 8: Seater; 9: Waste chamber; 10: Motor for beater; 11: Delivery pipe; 12: Exhaust air pipe.

each other for best results. The pair of feed rollers ensures a controlled feed of the tufts.

The grid is equipped with adjustable sheet metal guide slates interposed between the eight knife bars to control the passage of material. The strongly constructed grid with finished surfaces to which fibres cannot adhere is equipped with a simple four point suspension arrangement. They can be adjusted from outside in the graduated lever and brought into the proper position relative to the opening roller. It is thus possible to adjust the amount of waste and its quality to the requirements and the different types of raw materials.

The beater is equipped with toothed discs or saw tooth wire, and is suited to the technological requirements and the density of the opened material. Gentle handling and the highest possible degree of opening and cleaning of the fibres is thus achieved.

WORKING OF BEATERS

Type	Appearance	Description
Rollers	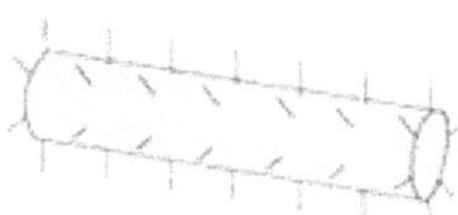	Small diameter, widely used, e.g. in step cleaners.
Drums	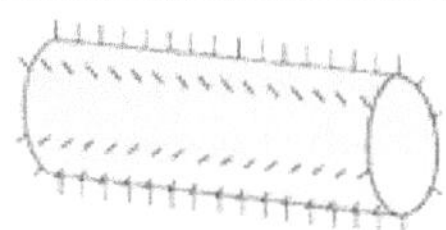	Larger diameter, e.g. in the mono-cylinder cleaner.
Quilted shaft	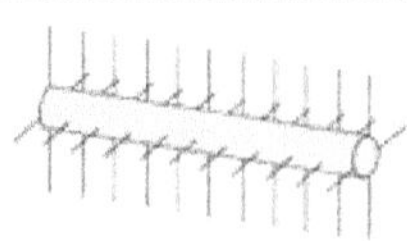	Shaft with many long beater rods, hardly used.
Multiple-bla-des beater	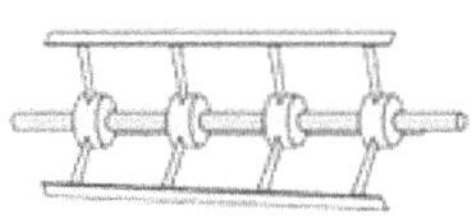	Two, three, or more arms. Now used only in old blowroom lines.
Spiked lattice	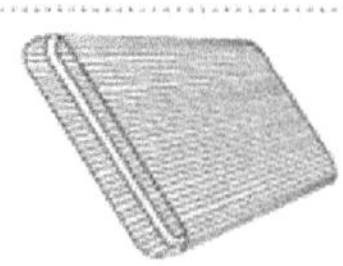	Endless belts with transverse woo-den or plastic bars in which needles are set, gives very gentle opening.
Picker	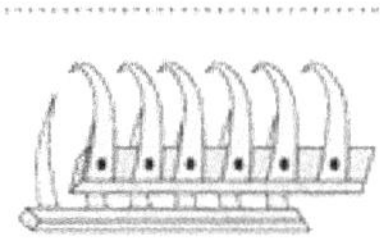	In the bale picker and blending grab (both outdated).
Carding bars or plates	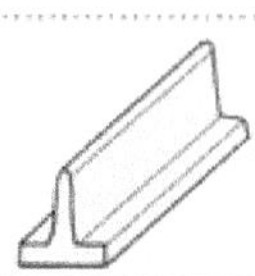	The devices associated with the carding drums of the card.

Figure 2.7: Opening Elements.

Porcupine Opener

This is very popular conventional opener suitable for all types of cotton with necessary modifications. This is a semi fast feeding bladed beater.

The cotton is fed on to the lattice A passing under pressure roller B to the fluted feed roller C which in conjunction with the pedal levers D holds the cotton while it is struck by the beater L. A grid bar system E is provided beneath the beater and as the cotton is detached from the grip of the feed system, It is impelled over the bars by the beater. The grid bars are usually triangular in section presenting a fairly sharp edge to the oncoming cotton and combined with the centrifugal action of the beater, they, effect the extraction of unwanted trash, which falls into the 'dead' air box F. A stripping rail G deflects the air stream and the cotton carried upon it into the passage H, at the upper end of which rotary screens or cages I are located. The cages, being connected to the fan J permit the dust-laden sir to pass thorough the perforations retain the cleaned lint on their surface in the form of a fleece, which is stripped by the delivery rollers K and deposited into the mouth pieces of a pipe line or onto the feed lattice of subsequent machine, according to requirements.

The extent and control of the air-flow through the opener has a considerable effect on the droppings of trash extraction. Air is admitted through adjustable vents M, tangentially to the rotating beater, just above the beating pint at roller C, insufficient quantity to keep the air flow at a speed which, while permitting trash particulars to escape through the bars E, will convey the more buoyant cotton to the cage I. Facilities are often provided to admit a small intake of the air into the trash box and so through the grid bars E, since in certain cases, s dead air box can make the dropping too 'rich' in spinnable fibre. Alterations to fan speeds are often made to attain a balance with the minimum of fibre loss.

Beater

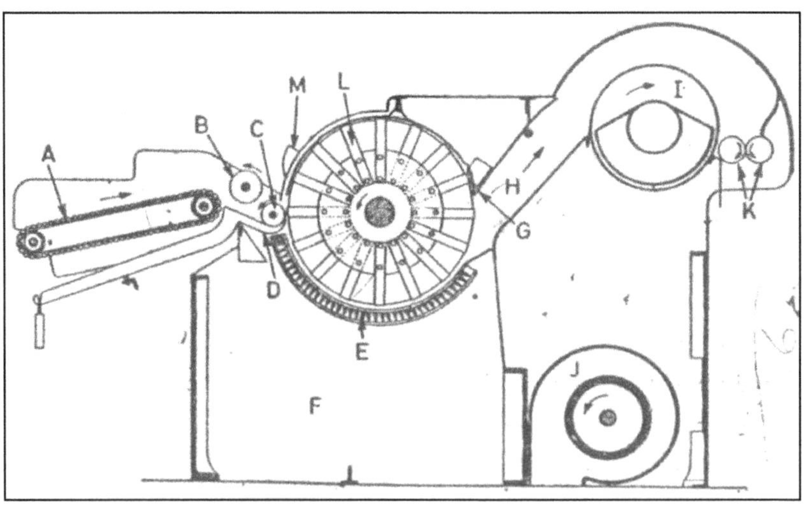

Figure 2.8: Porcupine Opener.

Figure A: Feed lattice; B: Pressure roller; C: Feed roller; D: Pedal lever: E: Grid bars; F: Dead air box; G: Stripping roll; H: Delivery passage; I: Cage; J: Fan; K: Delivery rollers; L: Bladed strikers; M: Adjustable vent.

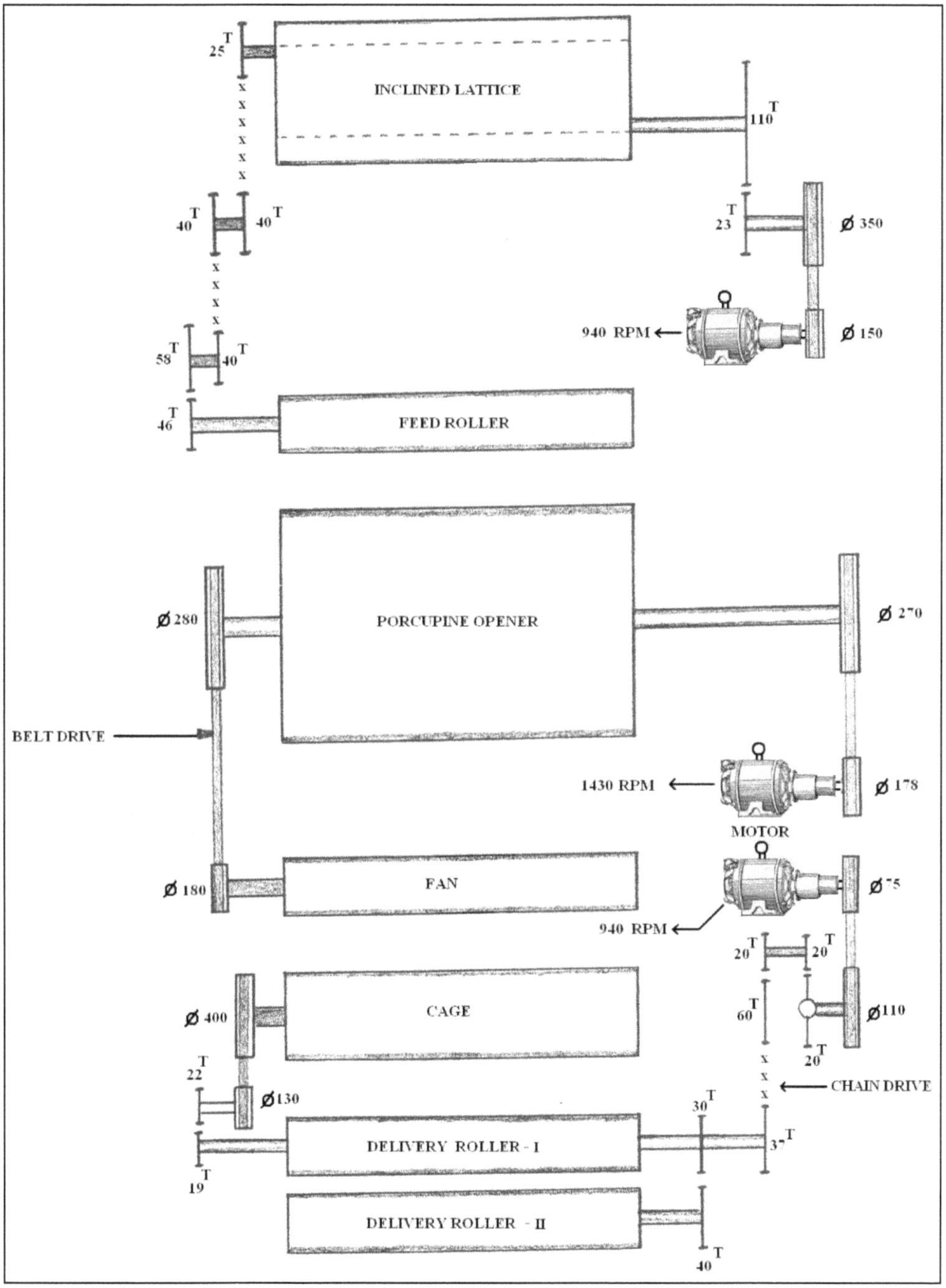

Figure 2.9: Porcupine Opener.

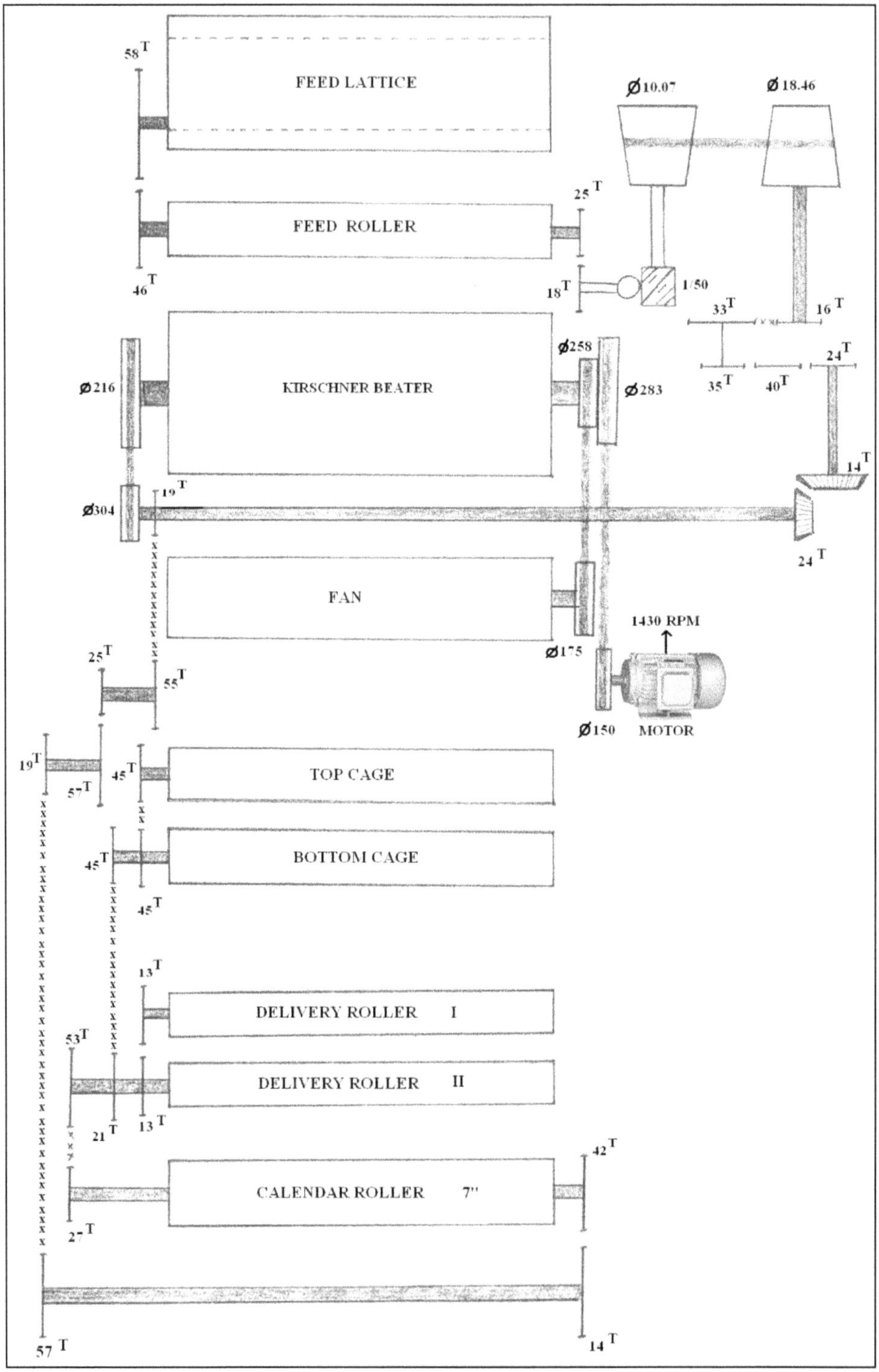

Figure 2.10: Kirschner Beater.

The principal feature of opening machine is the beater, which consists of upto sixteen circular discs, keyed onto a shaft and spaced apart by filling-in spacers, which prevent the cotton from getting between the discs and wound around the shaft. Riveted to the discs are projecting fingers or strikers 14 per discs for a 24" dia. Cylinder and 18 per disc for a 40" diameter cylinder-which act as the beating elements. These strikers are bent t various angles so that they do not track one behind another and they are arranged so that the whole width of the feed system in covered in one revolution of the beater.

PROCESS PARAMETERS

1. Number of Beating Points

The number of beating points (no. of blow room machines) depends upon the fibre parameters like Maturity, Fineness and Trash level of the cotton. More number of beating points or aggressive opening will lead to higher nep generation and fibre rupture. For example, for DCH Cotton, 1.5 Beating Point is enough and for Cotton like J34, the beating point varies 2.5 Beating Point because of higher trash content.

2. Beater Speed

Higher beater speed again lead to higher nep generation and fiber rupture. For Indian Cotton, Beater Speed 450to 600RPM works well.

3. Types of Beater

Proper design of the preparatory line and regular condition monitoring of the beaters is key to consistent yarn quality and good fibre yield. Fibre opening is key to good yarn spinning. Good, gentle opening ensures maximum retention of fibre strength by minimizing fibre rupture, reducing the level of neps, effective trash removal and minimal amounts of micro dust and lint.

In modern blow rooms, four types of beaters are primarily used - disc beaters, peg beaters, pinned beaters and saw tooth beaters, each having its own function and suitability to certain requirements and conditions. As disc and peg beaters are used exclusively for beating and pre-opening of cotton fibres.

It was not until the 1960s that blow room cleaning machines embraced metallic wire as an option to bladed, porcupine, vertical or pin beaters. Production limitations of traditional blow room lines of around 300 kg/hr gave way to metallic wire wound cylinders enabling dramatic increases in production. This provided more intense opening and cleaning, however, not without quality concession. Metallic wire in many applications results in fibre damage and requires frequent maintenance.

Typical Indian mills producing fine ring spun yarn up to the 1980s used up to seven cleaning points in their blow room lines and no metallic wire was used. Though in modern blow room lines, it is claimed that less cleaning points are required which helps reduce fibre damage at high productions rates, what is actually done is that multiple cleaning points are provided in a single blow room beater or card. However, even if one or two cleaning points are actually reduced, use of metallic wire leads to aggressive opening and consequent fibre rupture, which affects ring spun fine yarns quality in particular.

It may be prudent to replace the wire wound rolls with pinned rolls to reduce fibre damage, particularly for fine count, ring spun applications. Most super high production lines are suited for Open End Spinning operations where quality demands are more forgiving. Ring spun yarns, on the other hand, are very sensitive to speed, over beating, and aggressive cleaning. Machine makers are thus increasingly adopting the pin technologies to overcome some of the issues posed by aggressive metallic wire cleaning.

Engineering improvements, such as use of long lasting alloy steel pins, extruded alloy aluminum lags and special pin profiles, along with proven advanced methods of pin fixing that provides pin-point accuracy, have dramatically improved the performance of pinned beaters, which was never achieved in wooden products. The advantages of pinned beaters are:

- ☆ Pins provide extended product life.
- ☆ Pins are kind to fibres - reduced fibre rupture leading to yarn strength improvements.
- ☆ Pins provide fibre process flexibility.
- ☆ Pinned products are easily repairable (cost savings).
- ☆ Extruded aluminum tubes and profiles are lightweight alternatives of most metallic wire applications with cast or steel base rollers.
- ☆ High tech pin fixing methods provide pin point accuracy without grinding.
- ☆ Pin designs provide improved fibre transfer / doffing.

Choice of beaters and sequence of opening depends on the nature of fibre and the process requirements. Long staple cotton with low trash would require lesser beating and more opening than short staple, trashy cotton. Synthetic fibres require no beating and only gentle opening. Though not preferred, saw tooth wires can be used for opening polyester or nylon fibres. However, they can cause several problems if used for opening soft fibres like viscose since such fibres have a tendency to disintegrate under stress.

In saw tooth wire, the opening action is done by the knife-edges of the saw tooth, which tend to cut open the fibres (Figure 2.11). This leads to fibre rupture and lint generation. This tends to increase the percentage of short fibres and the level of neps. The trash contained in the fibre supply also tends to disintegrate into micro dust due to the saw tooth action.

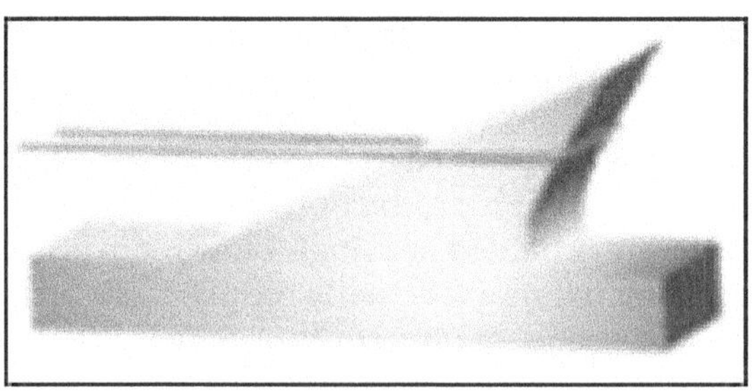

Figure 2.11: Action of Saw Tooth Wire.

In comparison, the pin has a smooth round surface and a spherical tip, which opens the fibres through a gentle untangling action (Figure 2.12). It is obvious that fibre rupture would be minimized as well as the consequent generation of micro dust and lint would also be reduced considerably with the use of pins. The round profile of pins also has another significant advantage - that of higher performing life and more consistent quality of opening.

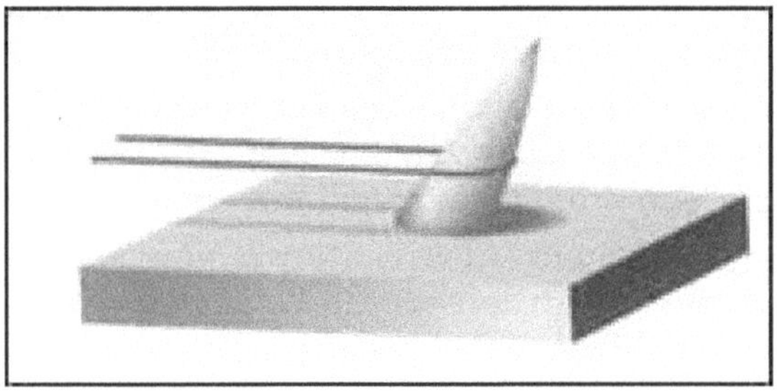

Figure 2.12: Action of Pinned Wire.

As the life time of saw tooth beater increases, the knife-edge gets rounded thus reducing opening action significantly. Moreover, small cuts or crevices develop on the leading edge of the saw tooth, which tends to 'Catch' the fibres and create neps. Usually, the edge of the saw tooth loses its sharpness in the first few months itself, thus causing a rapid deterioration in the fibre opening action. This is partially mitigated by grinding the roller so that the teeth regain their sharpness, but this lasts for much less duration before the deterioration occurs again.

Another significant effect of this loss of sharp edge is that the saw tooth begins to push fibres rather than open and carry them forward. This obviously results in an increase in fibre rupture, leading to a loss of rich fibre and lowering of fibre yield.

Since the pin has a rounded tip, it retains its opening ability much longer. Additionally, the wear all around the tip causes a new tip to be formed as the old one is eroded, though the pin length gets slightly reduced. This results in several significant benefits - increase in life of pins, more consistent opening action, thus ensuring a consistent sliver quality and a higher fibre yield as compared to saw tooth wires.

Key process conditions and requirements influencing selection of beater designs are:

a) Type of fibre - As mentioned earlier, synthetic fibres need to be opened using a different process than cotton. Even the type of cotton or synthetic fibres has a bearing on the preparatory process.

b) Cleaning - The percentage of trash in cotton will determine how many opening points and what intensity of beating are required.

c) Fibre rupture - There is a trade-off between better cleaning and fibre rupture so a delicate balancing act is required. What achieves better cleaning can also cause higher fibre rupture, if not carefully managed.

d) Micro dust - Saw tooth beaters are generally easier to use but in case of trash content being high, micro dust generation can be a problem with such beaters.

e) Lint - Low micronaire cotton tends to generate more lint with saw tooth wires.

f) Neps - Generally, neps level tends to increase with the increase in short fibre percentage, though this is not always the case. The preparatory system design has to consider the causes of neps to minimize them.

g) Production rate - What works in a low production line may not do so for high production rate. Consistency of quality becomes a primary factor when designing a high production preparatory line.

h) Desired quality of yarn — Preparatory requirements differ for fine counts and coarse counts, with fibre rupture being a much more significant quality factor in case of higher counts as is the levels of lint and neps.

i) Maintenance cost - This becomes a very sensitive issue in high production lines as breakdowns, repairs and reconditioning mean loss of production, increase in operating expenses and inconsistent quality.

j) Fibre yield - Sometimes there is a trade-off between higher fibre yield and a better-opened and cleaned fibre - which one is more important depends on the quality of yarn produced.

Design Factors in Beaters

1. Diameter - Increase in diameter helps reduce the rpm of the beater and also helps increase production. This is an option open only to machine manufacturers, though.
2. Opening points density; Projection and angle of points; and tip profile - they influence intensity of opening and cleaning, operating life, reduction in neps and fibre rupture.
3. Beater to Feed Roller Setting – Wider setting results in lesser Rupture and also less fibre Opening.
4. Beater to Grid Setting – The influence of this setting on fibre rupture is less. But too closer setting (Grid setting of 1) will lead to fibre rupture.
5. Fan Speed – it is advisable to run the fans at optimum speeds. Higher fan speeds will increase the material velocity and will create turbulence in the bends. This will result in curly fibres which will lead to entanglements. The influence of ventilator fan speed of material transport is lesser. But too high fan speed lead to higher fibre rupture.

4. PROCEDURE

1. Draw the complete gearing diagram of the machine
2. Show by arrow the flow of motion starting from motor to various parts
3. Mark various change pulleys / gears

4. Note down the diameters of the pulleys number of teeth of the gears and number of rows of spikes on evener roller.
5. List the various setting points.

5. CALCULATIONS

1. Calculate the rotational speeds of feed roller, beater, delivery roller, cages and fan in RPM and tabulate the results.

6. RESULTS

Tabulate the results.

	Feed Roller	*Beater*	*Delivery Roller*	*Cages*	*Fan Speed*
Rotational speed					
Surface speed					

3

Determination of the Intensity of Beating of Bladed Beaters and the Openness of Tufts and Cleaning Intensity

1. AIM

- ☆ To draw the gearing diagram of the machine
- ☆ To observe the design features and important functional elements of the machine / mechanism
- ☆ To calculate the speed of moving elements and Production of the machine in Kgs / Shift.
- ☆ To calculate the intensity of beating of beaters.
- ☆ To calculate the density of fibre after opening at each stage.

2. FORMULA

Refer spinning useful formula relevant to your experiment

3. DESCRIPTION

Raw cotton contains various kinds of trash, such as leaf, bark, and seed coat particles. The content of each of those trash categories is highly depending on the origin of the cotton and its harvesting method. Trash content from bale to silver should decrease through the opening. In one hand, the requirements of sliver quality impose that the cotton must be intensively cleaned during ginning, spinning mill and carding. On the other hand, the amount of those contaminations provides useful information for finding more efficient cleaning processes and predicts the quality of the finished products.

Opening is usually the first step in the spinning process and includes removal of the fibres from the bale by plucking followed by further opening using pinned cylinders and pinned lift aprons. Opening to a fine degree is normally performed using a feed roll/feed plate combination to restrain the cotton whilst it is opened into very small tufts by wire wound cylinders, pinned beaters or blade beaters. At each stage of opening a cleaning operation can be performed. Cotton has to be opened more than once because trash is removed only from the surface of tufts and multiple opening actions are needed to expose all the trash. In the blow room cotton tuft size vary from 5 mg to not more than 150 mg. Throughout the processing steps in the spinning plant the density of the fibre assembly changes in the following way:

Processing Step	*Density*
In the bale	0.30 – 0.70 g/cm^3
In mixer or blender	0.10 g/cm^3
In the sliver can	0.10 g/cm^3
On the roving bobbin	0.25 – 0.35 g/cm^3
Yarn on the bobbin	0.50 g/cm^3

Well-cleaned cotton enables the spinner to,

- ✩ Minimize ends down in spinning,
- ✩ Reduce the weak places caused by trash in the yarn,
- ✩ Spin fine yarns,
- ✩ Produce a more uniform yarn and fabric,
- ✩ Obtain a clean yarn and fabric,
- ✩ Improve downstream processing efficiencies.

Factors Influencing Cleaning in Blow Room

Normally trash is separated from the cotton by centrifugal force. The material is moved at high speed in a circular motion. The trash tends to sling out from the fibre surface during the passage in the pipe line. Grid bars are provided in the machines to allow the trash to escape and separate from the fibre that passes over the grid bars. The grid bars are adjustable to vary the angle and open space allowing more, or less trash to be removed. With an increase in the grid bar opening, there is an increase in the amount of good fibre that goes into the waste with the trash. Good fibre in the waste is normally kept to a minimal amount. However, if maximum cleaning is required there will be good fibre in the waste.

New tuft surfaces must be created continuously to facilitate cleaning. Larger, heavier particles are relatively easy to remove. Beating devices tend to break large trash particles making them smaller and more difficult to remove. Large trash should be removed at the beginning of the cleaning process. For this reason, cotton removed from the bales should be in small tufts for effective cleaning. Very small trash particles tend to be carried with the cotton in the transport air and it is difficult to obtain separation. Condensers and fibre separators help with the removal of dust sized particles.

Degree of Cleaning in the Blow Room

The trash content of cotton varies greatly, from 1% to as high as 15%. It is much more difficult to remove trash from cleaner cotton than it is from dirty cotton. The following table shows how much trash is normally removed from cotton with different trash levels.

Original Trash Content	*Quantity of Trash Removed*
$< 1.2\%$	$<40\%$
1.3 – 2.0%	40 – 50%
2.1 – 4.0%	50 – 60%
4.1 – 7.0%	55 – 65%
$\geq 7.1\%$	60 – 75%

As mentioned above some good fibre is lost with the trash. The appearance of the waste indicates the selectivity of the cleaning machine. The cleaning machines have to be carefully set to avoid excessive loss of good fibre but yet obtain the necessary trash removal action. An analysis of the waste using the Shirley Analyzer can give an objective measurement of the amount of good fibre in the waste. This can be expressed as a percentage of the waste material or as a percentage of the total material fed.

Definition to be Used

1. "Degree of Cleaning" - The numerical evaluation of the cleaning effect of a machine in spinning preparation is generally effected by detailing the degree of cleaning, which indicates in percentage terms the quantity of trash removal relative to the trash content present in the feed material.

$$\text{Degree of cleaning} = \frac{\text{Trash in input material} - \text{Trash in output material}}{\text{Trash in input material}} \times 100$$

2. "Cleaning Efficiency" – Refers to the percentage of trash contained in the waste removed by a cleaning machine. Low fibre content in the waste gives a high cleaning efficiency

$$\text{Cleaning efficiency} = \frac{\text{Total waste percentage} - \text{Fibre content percentage}}{\text{Total waste percentage}} \times 100$$

According to Zellweger USTER, the degree of cleaning DC, can be classified as follows:

Table 3.1: Classification of DC (%) for the Blow Room

Class	*Interpretation*
>40%	Very good
30 – 40%	Good
20 – 30%	Average
10 – 20%	Bad
<10%	Very bad

Table 3.2: Classification of DC (%) for the Card

Class	*Interpretation*
>90%	Very good
80 – 90%	Good
70 – 80%	Average
60 – 70%	Bad
<60%	Very bad

The degree of cleaning is influenced not only by the lint characteristics in intermediate products, but also by the mechanical handling of the fibre, because cotton has a lower degree of cleaning DC (%) if it is difficult to clean (bad cleanability) and/or if the machine has a lower cleaning efficiency. However, the degree of cleaning DC (%) is improved when the cotton is easy to clean (good cleanability) and/or when the cleaning efficiency of the machine is improved.

Determination of the Cleanability

In order to get meaningful results of cleaning efficiency, it is important to know the behaviour of the cotton to cleaning; it is the easiness or the difficulty with which cotton is rid of its trash. Several methods are used to determine the cleanability C. The most simple consist to determine the relationship between the percentage of trash eliminated after one passage T1 of the sample in the control device Micro Dust Trash Analyzer, MDTA3, and T_{total} of this same sample. C-factor depends on successive passages of the control device 'Uster-MDTA 3', more the quantity of trash T1 collected in the first passage is raised more the cleanability of cotton is better.

Leifeild developed a systematic, mathematical description of the various factors effects upon cleaning efficiency, with the objective of being able to predict the results of cleaning processes and proposed the following empirical formula:

$$Dc\ (\%) = 10 \times C \times T_{total} \times M_{cl}$$

where,

Dc (%) = degree of cleaning

M_{cl} = cleaning efficiency (represents the influence of the machine)

T_{total} = trash content

C = cleanability of the cotton. A high C factor means good cleanability, a low C-factor characterizes cotton that is difficult to clean.

BLADED BEATERS

The *intensity of opening* is a fundamental factor above all in this stage, as it is necessary to disentangle the tufts and eliminate foreign matter, but at the same time any damage to the very delicate fibre must be prevented. This depends essentially on the following conditions:

1. T*he opener feeding system,* which can be:
   a. *free mass* when the tufts driven by the air flow come into contact with the cylinder rods, without being retained by feeding devices;
   b. *in laps* when the tufts, on passing from the cleaner cylinder rules are retained by an apron (on the right of the diagram) and a feeder cylinder, and are delivered in the form of laps; the lap feeder can be either vertical or horizontal. In the first case, the tufts escape the action of the rods after having received just one beat; in the second case, after the first beat, the tuft rebounds on the grid and comes once again into contact with the cylinder rods, that beat it further. The vertical lap feed provides a higher degree of opening;
2. The *rods section,* that can be flat or round: the first type have a stronger hold on the tufts and therefore offer a higher degree of opening, but they risk de-fibrating the fibres even more; the above mentioned action is increased if the rods are sharp;
3. The *angular speed of the cylinder,* as this determines the number of beats that the fibre is subject to and the centrifugal force that they undergo as an effect of the rod beatings;
4. The *distance between the grid and the cylinder rods*: in fact with the minimum distance between them the highest degree of opening is achieved, as the tufts hit the grid at the top speed;
5. The *distance between the small bars of the grid,* which can be varied by rotating the bars on their longitudinal axis by a lever or a wheel: reducing the distance between the bars reduces the degree of opening and cleaning;
6. The *distance between the feeder cylinders and the cylinder rods,* which depend on the average length of the cotton being processed, generally this distance must increase proportionally to the length of the fibre, as the latter could get ruined or break under the beats from the rules;
7. *The air flow*: varying the air flow that accompanies the fibre during the processing cycle, the time the cotton remains in the machine changes and therefore so does the degree of opening.

1. Three Bladed Beater

This is a semi fast feeding bladed beaters and mostly employed after sufficient preliminary opening. The outstanding feature of the beater is that each blade strikes the fringe of cotton delivered by the feed system simultaneously so that nothing

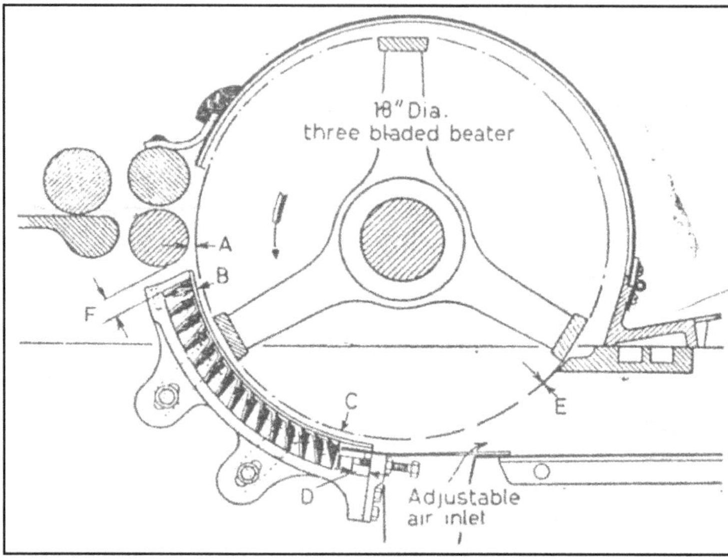

Figure 3.1: Three Blade Beater.

1: Pedel and pedel roller; 2: Pair of feed rollers; 3: Adjustable grid bar system; 4: Three bladed beater; 5: Leathed flap cover; 6: Stripping rajj; 7: Adjustable air inlet.

within that fringe can dodge the blow, and it is particularly noticeable that the bladed beater is most effective in extracting motes, which have fibre attached and so tend to evade other types of strike beater.

The blades running across the width of the machine are made of steel, and are firmly riveted to three or four sets of arms keyed on the shaft. Each edge of the blade is beveled in order to strike the cotton clearly. The amount of the bevel is not however sufficient to have a cutting action on the emerging cotton, as the edge is dulled through continnal usage, it is now usual to reverse the beater. When this happens, both ends of the shaft being made alike for this purpose, this brings the other beveled edge of the blade into use.

The rapidly repeated blows striking, the cotton away in small tufts and dashing them against grid bars covering one fourth of the circumference of the beater, starting near of the feed, the dirt is driven out between them and falls into a suitable chamber.

Settings

A – The settings between the beater and feed roller

B – The setting between the beater and the first grid bar

C - The setting between the beater and the last grid bar

E - The setting between the stripping rail and the beater

F - The setting between the bottom of the feed roller to first grid bar.

A wider setting is mainly used for long-stapled cottons to prevent too severe treatment of the fringe. If a very heavy feed is used, the settings should be wider, so as

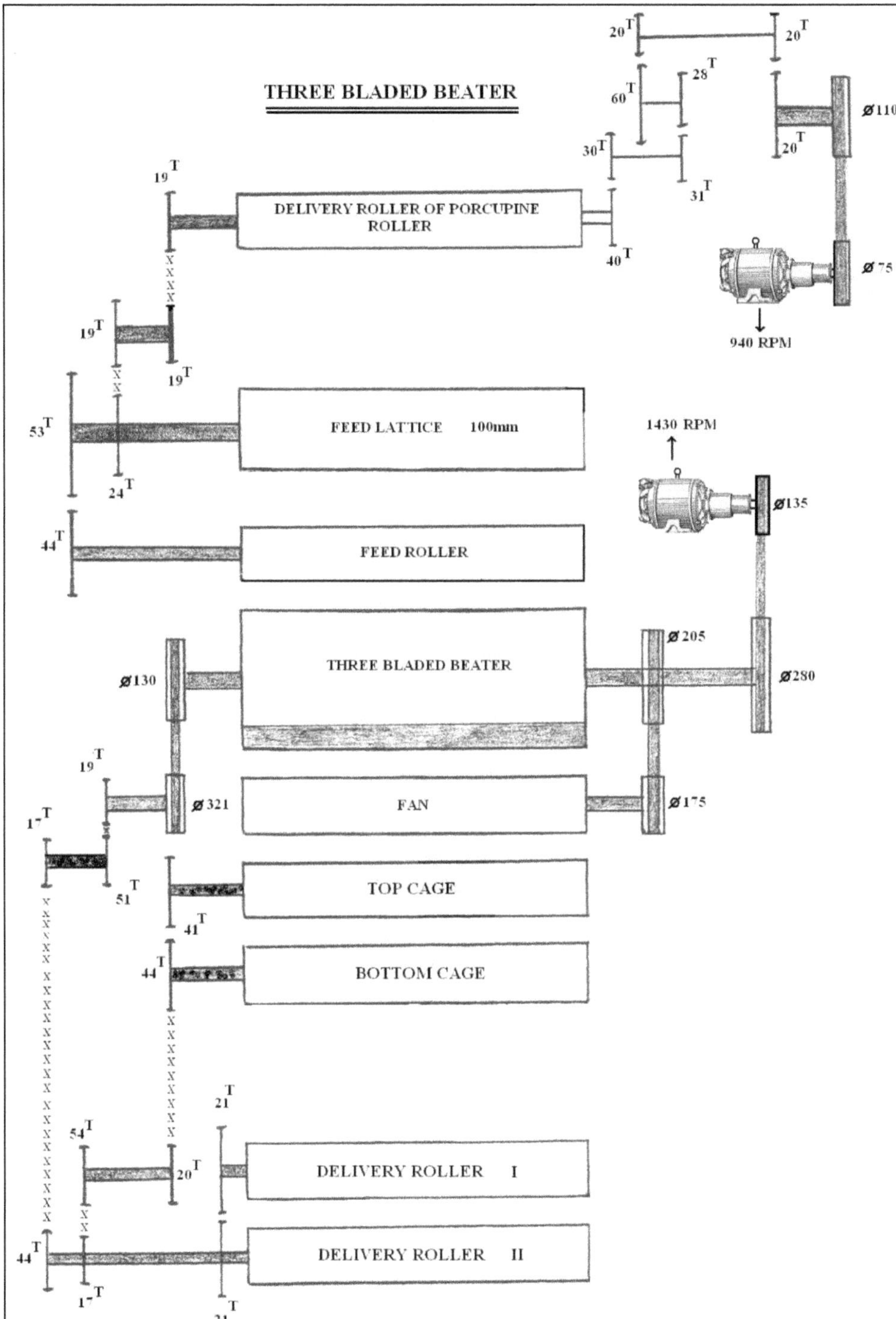

Figure 3.2: Three Bladed Beater.

not to crush the fibres too much between the beater and the feed roller or pedal, which would cause nep and broken fibre.

INTENSITY OF BEATING

It defines the number of blows / beats imparted to a unit length of material being fed by the feeding device of the beater. Mathematically,

Intensity of Beating = $N \times b / X$

where,

N = revolution of beater in rpm

b = Number of beater blades

X = length of material fed / min

Procedure

1. Draw the drive to the beater shaft and its feed system
2. Measure the diameter of various pulleys
3. Count the number of teeth of various gears
4. Measure the distance of the beater blade from the centre of the beater.

Calculations

1. Determine the speed of the beater shaft and feed rate (cm / min)
2. Find out the intensity of beating using the equation
3. Calculate the surface speed of the beater blade.

OPENNESS OF TUFTS

Openness value may be measured by determining the apparent specific volume of a collection of tufts.

$$\text{Apparent Specific volume} = \frac{\text{Sample (slightly compressed) Volume (cm}^3\text{)}}{\text{Sample Weight}}$$

For comparison between various types of fibres, openness value should be determined by the following formula:

Openness value = Apparent Sp. Vol. x Specific gravity the fibres

Procedure

1. Collect 100 gm of tufts from any point of blow room.
2. Remove tufts carefully from the sample and fill the beaker as uniformly as possible. Tufts should be seen against light so as to make sure that two tufts are not neither sandwiched nor buried in to each other.
3. Place the disc on the tufts and allow it to settle down for 30 sec.
4. Note down the height of the compressed tufts and inside diameter of the beaker.
5. Repeat the test for five times.

Calculation

1. Volume of the compressed sample = nD2h / 4

   Where D = diameter of the beaker

   h = height of the compressed sample
2. Apparent sp. Vol. as defined
3. Openness value (Sp. Gravity of Cotton = 1.54, Polyester = 1.32, Viscose rayon = 1.54)

6. RESULTS

Tabulate the results

Sl.No.	*Height of the Compressed Tufts*	*Beater dia*	*Sp. Vol*	*Openness Value*
1				
2				
3				
4				
Average				

4

Construction and Working Mechanism of Blending Machines

1. AIM

- ✰ To draw the motion transmission path of the blending machines.
- ✰ To observe the design features and important functional elements of the machine / mechanism.
- ✰ To calculate the speed of rotating elements, delivery rate in mpm, and Production of the machine in Kgs / Shift.

2. FORMULA

Refer spinning useful formula relevant to your experiment

3. DESCRIPTION

The Multiple Mixer MPM (Figure 4.1) is constructed with 6, 8, 10 or 12 hoppers each 50 mm long, depending upon the requirements for blending and capacity. The height of the hoppers is deduced from the overall height of the machines minus the 1500 mm height of the base unit which contains the delivery rollers, opening rollers and the blending channel. This blend is blown from the preceding machine by the material transport fan and conveyed into the feed duct above the hoppers. The conveyor air is ducted through perforated plates in the upper part of the hoppers into exhaust ducts on the side from there into the blending channel below the opening rollers. The hoppers are closed against the feed duct by pneumatically operated flaps, apart from the first hopper in the direction counter to the material flow.

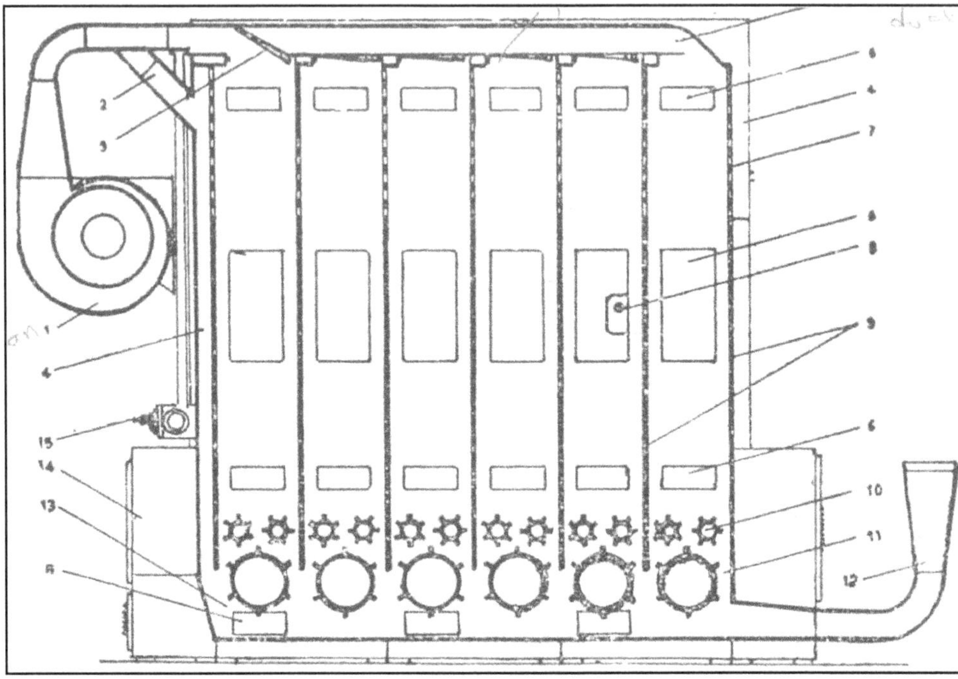

Figure 4.1: Multi Mixer.

1: Pan; 2: Air by-pass; 3: Filling flaps; 4: Exhaust duct; 5: Feed duct; 6: Inspection hatch; 7: Perforated sheet; 8: Photo cell; 9: Hopper wall; 10: Delivery roller; 11: Opening roller; 12: Suction funnel; 13: Blending channel; 14: Programme control; 15: Electronic pressure switch.

The charging of the multi mixer at the beginning of a blend lot starts with the first hopper at the end of the feed duct. It is filled only to just below the photocell situated in the adjacent hopper which governs the minimum charging level during automatic operation. Then the closing flap of the second hopper is opened by push button operation. The second hopper is charged to a rather higher than the second. The charge level of the hoppers raises uniformly up to the last hopper which is fully charged.

Whilst the last hopper is being charged there is a change-over to automatic operation and the material transport is switched on. The columns of material in the hoppers start to drop. When the last hopper is full the closing flap shuts automatically and charging restarts with the first hopper as soon as the level of the second hopper has dropped below the photocell.

The graduated charging levels of the hoppers are thus maintained during automatic operation. The last charged hopper is always situated adjacent to the hopper with the lowest charge. As all the hoppers are emptied simultaneously, fibres come together in the blending channels which have come from the preceding machine at different times.

When the charging level rises, more and more of the holes in the perforated plate of the upper part of the hopper are blocked with the material. This increases the pressure of the conveyor air. Once a preselected pressure is reached, which corresponds to the particular charging level, an electronic switch closes the flap of this hopper and opens up the flap of the next hopper. The pressure that is set for the changeover is displayed on a manometer. The capacity of the hoppers may be varied by altering the changeover pressure.

The base of each hopper is closed by a pair of delivery rollers which transfer the material gradually and uniformly, but without applying the pressure which might damage the fibres, to an opening roller with six toothed strips. the delivery rollers of all the hoppers are driven by two variable speed motors with a control range up to 1:6.

The opening rollers gently loosen the material into tufts and deliver them into the blending channel from which they are sucked by the subsequent condenser. The opening rollers of all the hoppers are driven by two 3-phase motors, the power of which conforms to the number and width of hoppers.

When the blend lot is changed the Multimixer must be emptied. The machine is reset to manual control before the entire batch has been evaluated in order to be able to take material from all the hoppers right up to the end of the batch. Operation is then switched to next hopper when charging level of the preceding hopper is reached.

UNIMIX

This machine is made up of three parts: storage section, an intermediate chamber and a delivery section (Figure 4.2).

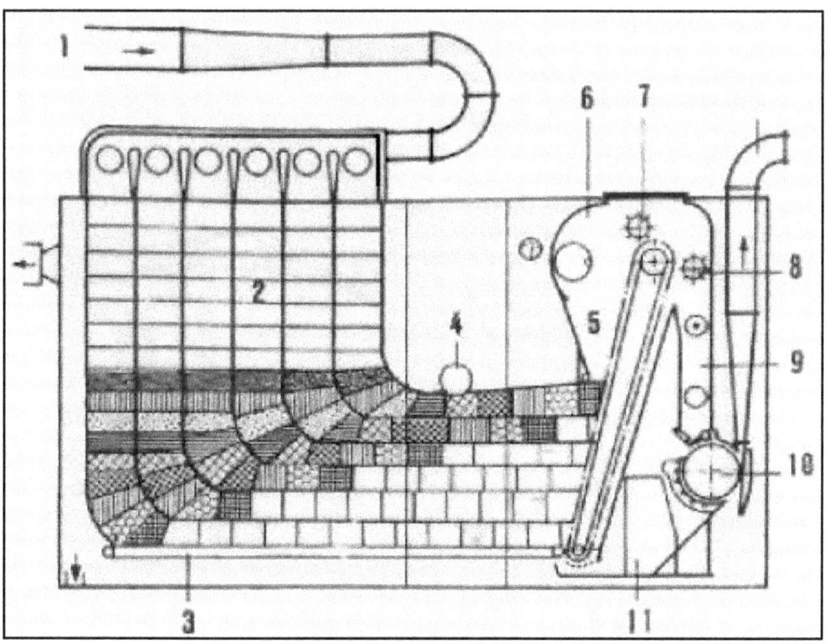

Figure 4.2: Unimix.

Flocks are fed pneumatically and simultaneously into six J-shaped chutes (2), arranged one behind the other in the storage section. A conveyor belt (3) leads the stock through the intermediate chamber to the take-off unit. The material columns are thus diverted out of the vertical in to the horizontal.

In addition to a condensing effect, this 90° bend in the material flow also produces a shift in the timing and spatial distribution of transport of the fiber packets from the first to the last chute. This in turn results in good long-term blending. Thereafter, as in a blending opener, material is extracted from the intermediate chamber and subjected to a further opening step between an inclined spiked lattice (5) and an ever roller (7), giving an additional good short-term blending.

An optical sensor ensures that only a small quanity of fibre stock is held in the mixing chamber (6). After the spiked lattice, there is either a simple pneumatic-suction feed to the next machine or a cleaning unit. Both blending and cleaning machines are thus provided in a single piece of equipment.

3-Point Blending

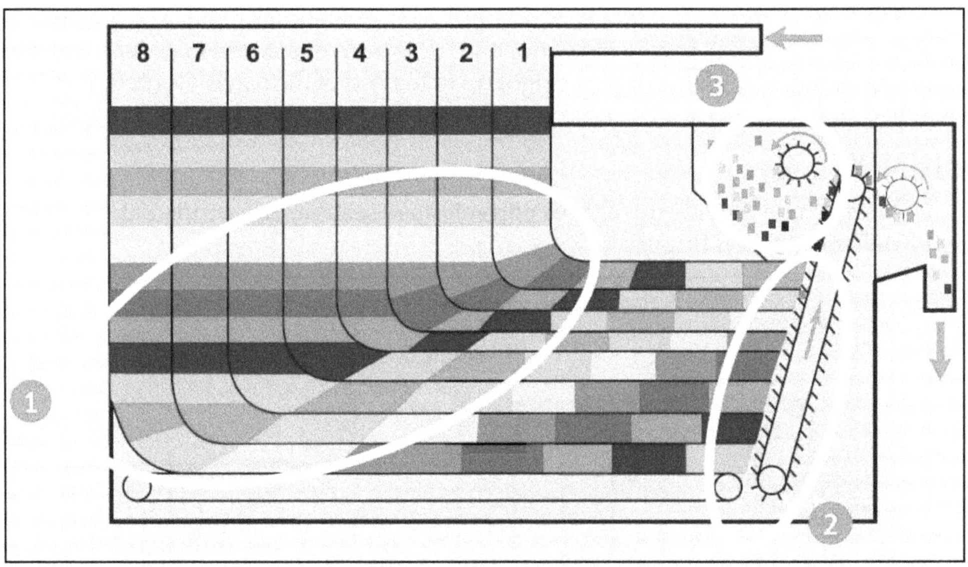

Figure 4.3: 3-Point Blending.

1. Deflection of the tuft mass through 90° in the UNImix displaces these layers in terms of space and time. The result is defined, long-term blending.
2. The spiked feed lattice removes tufts simultaneously from all 8 layers. This gentle separation process inevitably results in a second, thorough blending of the tufts. The blend is already homogeneous at this point.
3. A third, intensive mixing of the free tufts takes place in the opening roller zone. This additional, thorough blending ensures the constant homogeneity of the fiber blend.

UNIBLEND

The UNIblend A 81 has been specially designed for staple fibers.It is used to obtain a specific blend of widely-differing types of material.

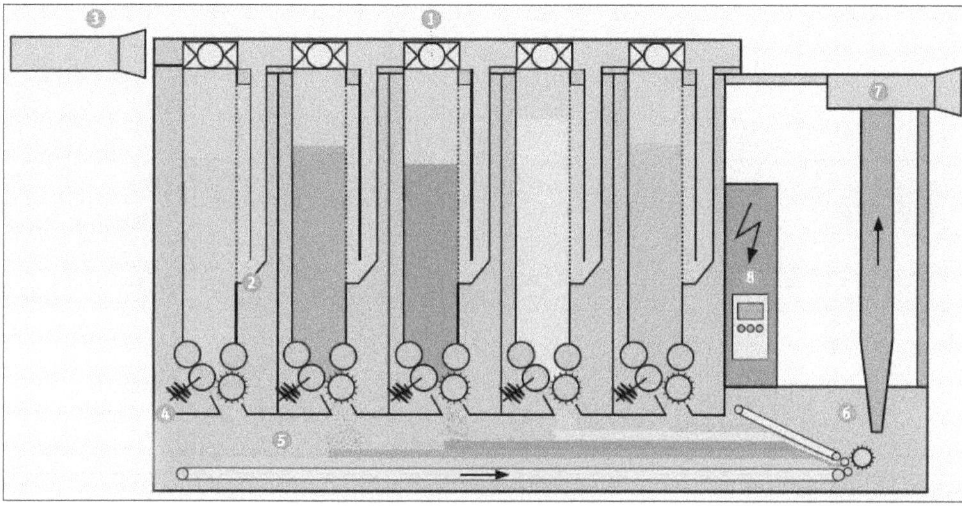

Figure 4.4: Uniblend.

1: Material feed; 2: Dedusting and air extraction; 3: Air to filter unit; 4: Dosage unit; 5: Component layers; 6: Take-off unit; 7: Inverter-controlled transport fan; 8: Control cabinet.

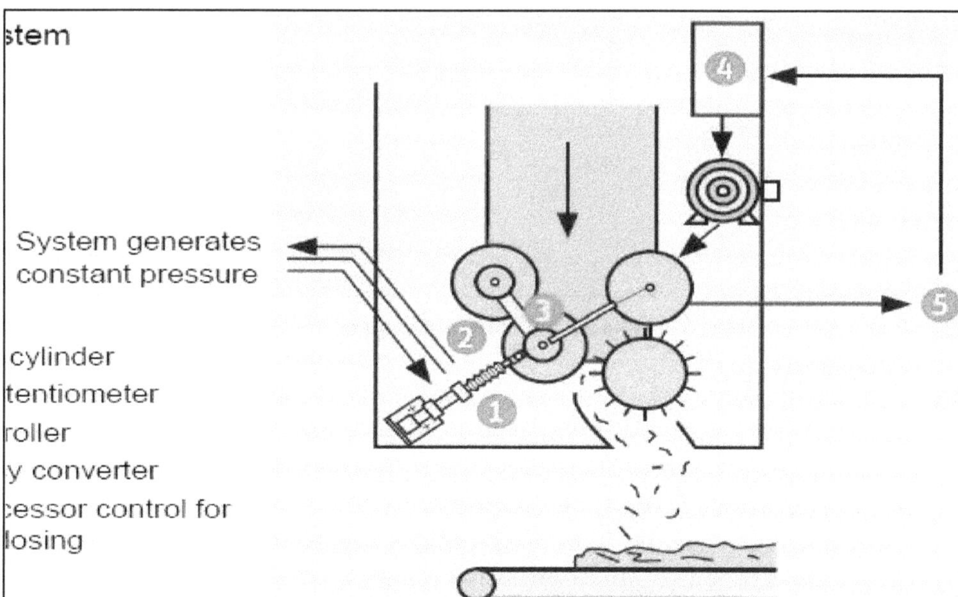

Figure 4.5: Dosgae System.

1: Pressure cylinder; 2: Linear potentiometer; 3: Opening roller; 4: Frequency converter; 5: Microprocessor control for constant dosing.

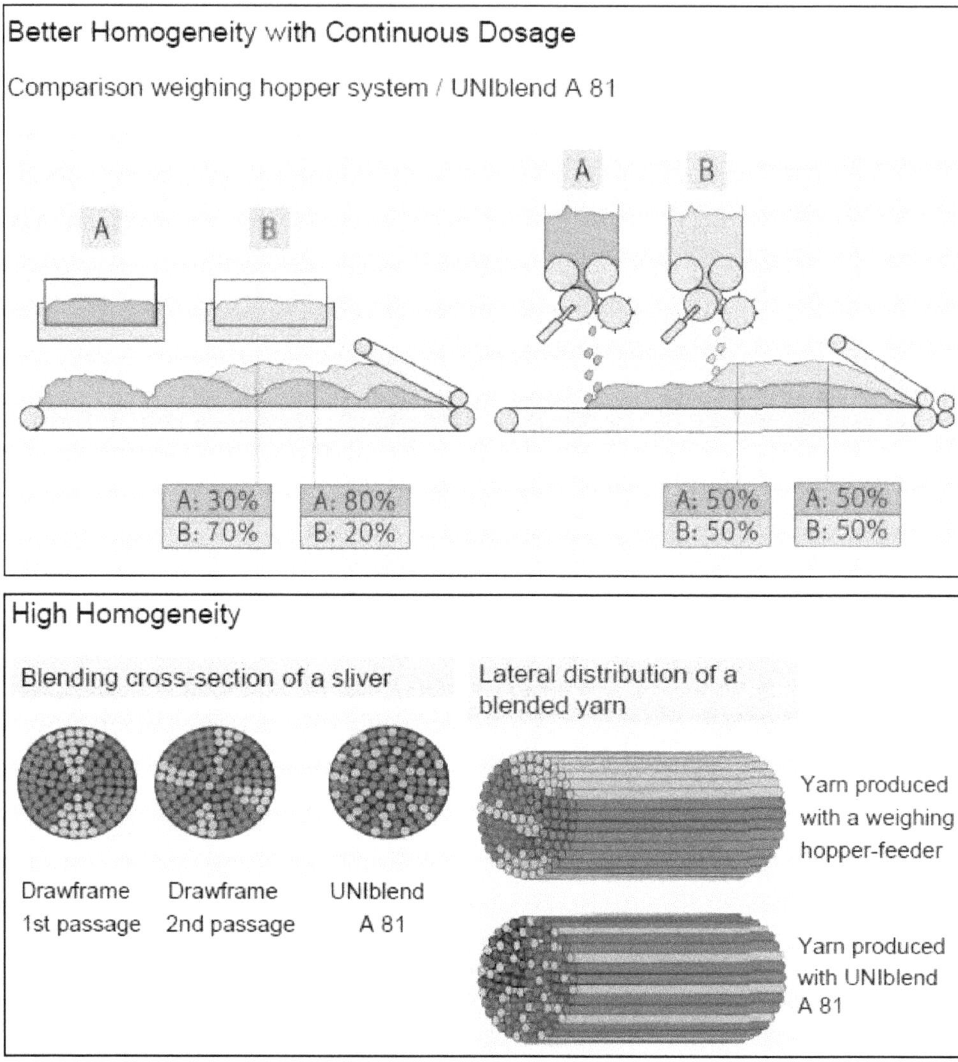

Figure 4.6: Blend Analysis.

4. PROCEDURE

1. Draw the complete gearing diagram of the machine
2. Show by arrow the flow of motion starting from motor to various parts
3. Mark various change pulleys / gears
4. Note down the diameters of the pulleys, number of teeth of the gears and number of rows of spikes on evener roller.
5. List the various setting points.

5. CALCULATIONS

1. Calculate the rotational speeds of feed roller, beater, conveyor, inclined lattice, evener roller in RPM and tabulate the results.

6. RESULTS

Tabulate the results

	Feed Roller	*Beater*	*Conveyor*	*Inclined Lattice*	*Evener Roller*
Rotational speed					
Surface speed					

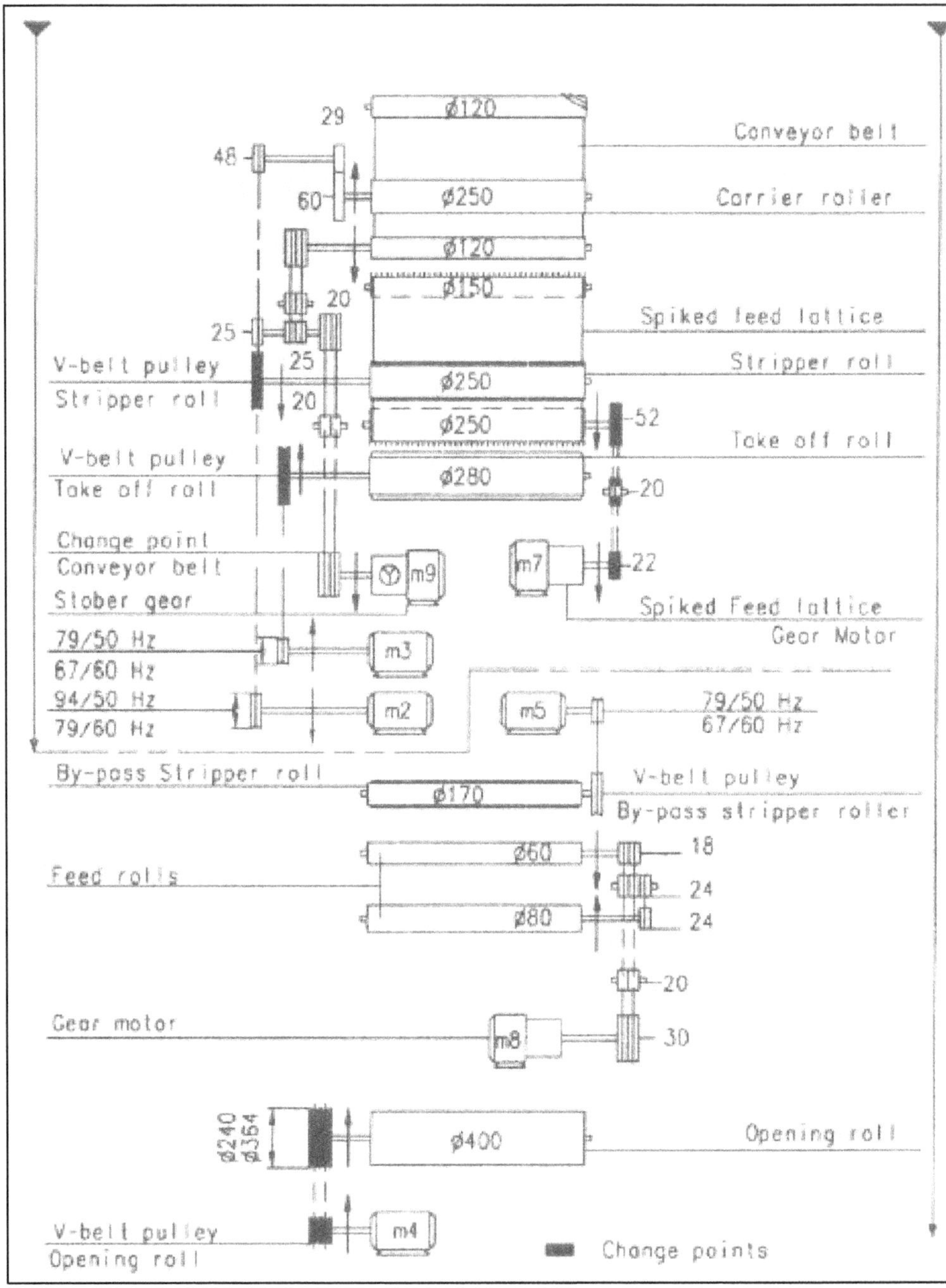

Figure 4.7: Cleaning Diagram of Unimix.

LAKSHMI	UM 01	Page 6	Issue No : 01	Rev.
			September 2003	Date

3.2 Speed chart , Fig. 4

Conveyor belt

Motor m9 * 50Hz/60hZ = 2.45 min^{-1}

Speed range m/min
0.14 – 1.00

* Inverter driven

Spiked feed lattice

Motor m7 * 50Hz/60hZ = 190 min^{-1}

Speed range m/min
20 - 100

* Inverter driven

Stripper roll

Motor m2 * Inverter driven

50 Hz, 1380 min^{-1} Motor pulley Ø 94		60 Hz, 1650 min^{-1} Motor pulley Ø 79	
Roller pulley	Rpm min^{-1}	Roller pulley	Rpm min^{-1}
Ø 144	887	Ø 144	884
Ø 174	731	Ø 174	728
Ø 216	586	Ø 216	584

Take-off roll

Motor m3

50 Hz, 1380 min^{-1} Motor pulley Ø 79		60 Hz, 1650 min^{-1} Motor pulley Ø 67	
Roller pulley	Rpm min^{-1}	Roller pulley	Rpm min^{-1}
Ø 136	784	Ø 134	788
Ø 154	690	Ø 154	693
Ø 194	545	Ø 194	547

By-pass roll

Motor m5

50 Hz, 930 min^{-1} Motor pulley Ø 79		60 Hz, 1115 min^{-1} Motor pulley Ø 67	
Roller pulley	Rpm min^{-1}	Roller pulley	Rpm min^{-1}
Ø 119	606	Ø 119	608

Opening roll

Motor m9 50Hz = 1430 min^{-1} 60Hz = 1716 min^{-1}

Motor pulley	Beater pulley	Roller rpm min^{-1}	
		50 Hz	60 Hz
Ø 89	Ø 240		618
Ø 104	Ø 240	606	
Ø 116	Ø 240		814
Ø 136	Ø 240	780	960
Ø 164	Ø 240	982	
Ø 104	Ø 364	397	

Feed rolls

Motor m8 * 50Hz/60Hz = 56 min^{-1}

Speed range m/min
1.2 – 18.8

* Inverter driven

Fig. 4

Figure 4.8: Details of Gearing Diagram.

5

Construction and Working Mechanism of Scutcher and Lap Forming Unit

1. AIM

- ☆ To draw the motion transmission path from motor to various parts of the scutchers unit
- ☆ To observe the design features and important functional elements of the machine / mechanism
- ☆ To calculate the speed of rotating elements, delivery rate in mpm, and Production of the machine in Kgs / Shift.

2. FORMULA

Refer spinning useful formula relevant to your experiment

3. DESCRIPTION

The objects of scutchers is to further break down tuft size, cleaning, by a beater section and to produce a uniform sheet of cotton both longitudinally and transversely to be wound in the form of a lap. To achieve the above objects the scutcher line consists of

- ☆ Automatic Hopper Feeder to receive cotton from the cleaning line
- ☆ Feed regulating motion
- ☆ Beater section
- ☆ Lap forming and Measuring motion.

CONVENTIONAL SCUTCHERS

Hopper Feeder

In a single process, the cotton is fed to the scutcher from the cleaning line through an Automatic Hopper Feeder. The principle object of the Hopper Feeder is to provide a uniform feed to the subsequent machine.

The sectional elevation (Figure 5.1) shows the salient features of an automatic hopper feeder. The reserve bin is fed by a condenser mounted above the bin. When the reserve bin is adequately filled with stock, the feeler plate is deflected which switches off the motor driving the spiked lattice of the preceding machine through relays. The reserve bin provides a simple means of keeping the level of stock in the main bin at a constant volume irrespective of the fluctuations in delivery of the preceding machine, by the bottom lattice in conjunction with the claw roller.

The regularity of the end product lap begins at this point because the volume of cotton contained in bin determines largely the amount of stock carried upwards by the spiked lattice which is influenced by the area of cotton presented to the spiked lattice and the pressure of cotton against the spikes due to the forward movement of the bottom lattice. The evener roller, removes the insufficiently opened excess cotton from the spikes of the elevating lattice which in turn stripped by the stripper roller into the bin for further treatment.

The main feature of automatic hopper feeder is the reserve delivery. The spiked lattice is extended to a much greater height than the ordinary hopper feeder. In order to achieve a larger stock and uniform density at the bottom of the chute, the back sheet hinged at K reciprocates, alternately compressing and releasing. This action combined

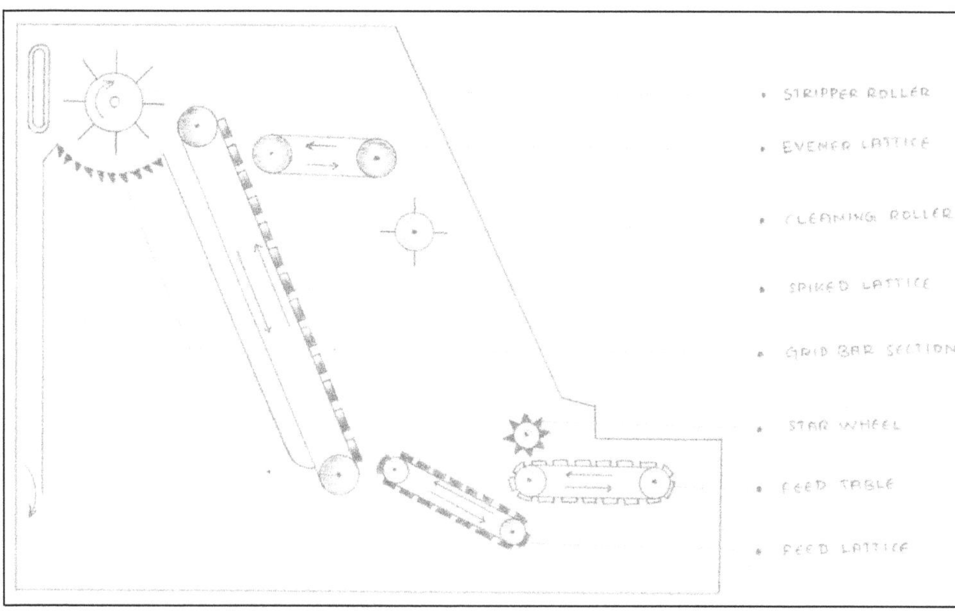

Figure 5.1: Hopper Feeder

with the constant head maintained by the return roller ensures the maximum regularity of feed to the scutcher.

Piano Feed Regulating Motion

The pedal movement caused by the thick and thin places of cotton is employed to shift the belt in the cone drums by means of levers to alter the speed of the feed roller in order to keep the feed constant per unit time.

To design a pair of cone drums which produce the requisite variation of feed roller speed to maintain a given quantity of cotton, it is assumed that the minimum thickness is ¼" and the maximum thickness of 1" with the bottom driving cone drum rotating at a constant speed of 100 rev / min. Uniform increments in the thickness of cotton passing between the feed roller and the pedal lever must be given uniform increments of movements to the belt along the cone drum. The cone drum belt shifting mechanism is connected to and receives its motion from the pedal levers, through the regulating motion.

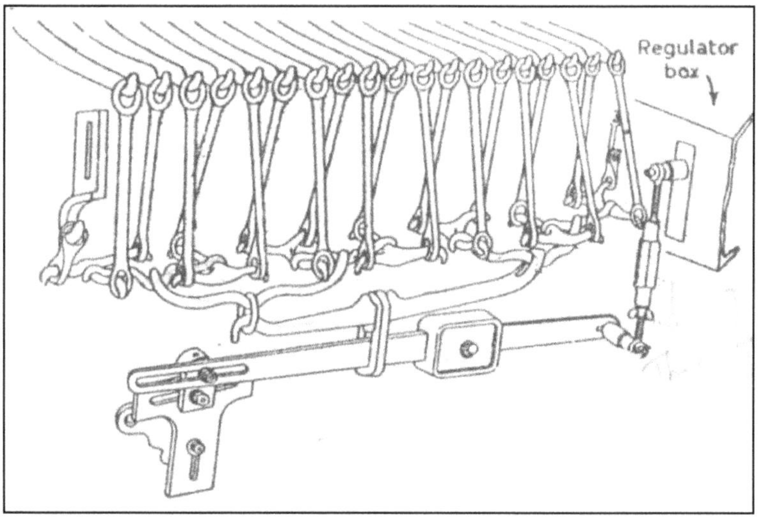

Figure 5.2: Piano Feed Motion.

The salient features of the mechanism are shown in figure. Eighteen pedal levers are placed side by side across the width of the machine and mounted on a knife edge rail to avoid friction. The variation in thickness of cotton at feed point is multiplied 5 to 6 times at the tail end of the lever, which is usually in the form of a hook. On the hooked end of each lever, in this system pendent links are provided. The pedal ends are linked up in sets of three to suitable tripod levers, which in turn are connected in pairs by simple levers down to the bottom long lever which in turn is connected to the belt fork mechanism in the cone drum box.

Each pedal detects its own section of approximately two inches, and the summation of the movement of the pedal levers, by means of the linkages, determines the amount of movements as the belt fork and so increases or decreases the top cone speed, which in turn drives the feed roller and lattice faster or slower to keep the feed uniform.

Opening Section

The objective of this section is to open the cotton further to small tuft size and to extract as much as possible of the trash remaining in the cotton making the lap for the card. Three types of beaters are commonly used

1. Porcupine beater
2. The bladed beater
3. Kirschner beater

Kirschner Beater

This is the semi-fast feeding pin opener. With improvements in trash extracting at earlier stages of processing, the extraction of trash at the scutcher has been of less importance than the making of a uniform well-textured lap.

It consists of 'Three Armed Spikes' mounted on a shaft, with wooden lags firmly fixed to the arms, each lag carries a large number of harded, well pointed, steel pins arranged in staggered from to ensure adequate combing of the cotton across the whole width of the machine. Further, there is a slight taper in the wooden lags when mounted, the leading edge being thinner than the trailing edge. This has a effect of a graduated penetration of cotton fringe at each blow of beater, minimizing any tendency to pluck uncombed tufts from the fringe. It is normally run at speeds around 700 to 750 rpm. This type of beater is not considered to be a good cleaning machine. But it produces a smooth and well opened sheet of cotton for the card.

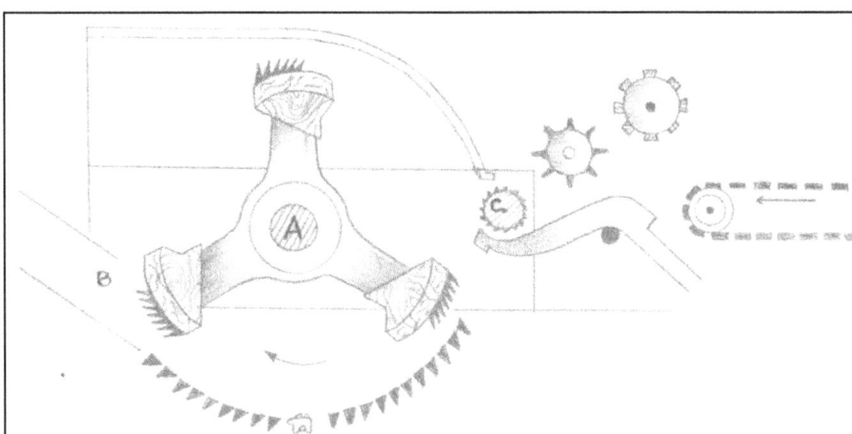

Figure 5.3: Kirschner Beater.
A: Beater; B: Stripping rail; C: Feed roller with pedal.

Condensing Cages

The condensing cages in the scutcher play a most important part in the uniform distribution of the opened and cleaned cotton, particularly across the width of the machine. The cages are made of either woven wire or perforated tinned sheets mounted on cast iron circles. The air flow, by which the cotton is conveyed from the beater to the cages, is induced by the fan situated beneath the cages and connected to them by air-flues from the end of each cage. The air, in passing through the perforations of the cages deposits uniform fleece of cotton on to their surfaces. In practice, however, mainly owing to lack of air control, faults occur, such as the formation of conical laps caused by the depositing of more cotton on one side than the other. Barrel shaped laps are due to excessive fan speed. The dust laden air exhausted by the fan is blown into a dust settling chamber.

Lap Forming

As the cotton leaves the cages, it is collected and lightly pressed by a pair of fluted delivery rollers, which have the same surface speed as the cages and it then passes on to the calendar rollers of the machine. There are four calendar rollers made of highly polished cast iron, mounted in suitable sides, one above the other and heavily weighted, a force of up to 2 tones being applied by means of levers. The cotton passes out between top and second calendar rollers and then leaves between bottom and third calendar rollers. After leaving the calendar rollers, the sheet of cotton passes beneath a 'dead' or pressure roller which helps to maintain the compacted condition of the sheet as it is delivered to the fluted shell rollers. Resting between the two shell rollers is the lap "pin" or lap roller, rotated by the shell rollers. The operative places the sheet between the lap pin and shell-roller and then applies pressure at each end of the pin.

Formation of Compact Lap

The pressure on the lap during the period of building up to the requisite weight is usually obtained by a suitable brake mechanism. In this arrangement, the racks mounted on suitable slides on the machine framing, engage the ends of the lap pin at B, where antifriction bearings are usually fitted. The lower ends of the racks are provided with teeth, which are geared into the pinions, gear C mounted on a cross

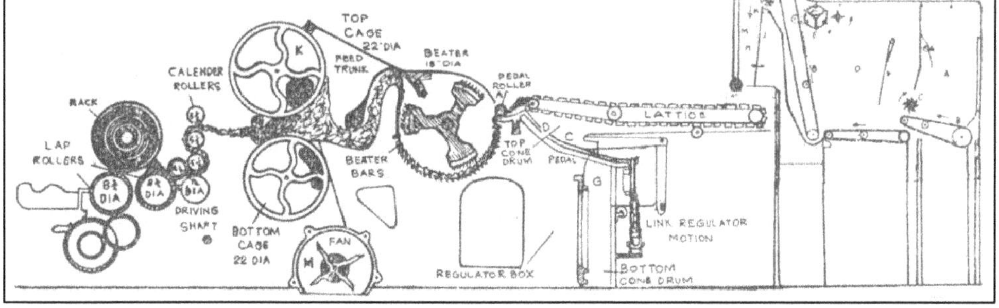

Figure 5.4: Scutecher and Hopper Feeder.

A: Reserve bin; B: Bottom lattice; C: Claw roller; D: Main bin; E: Evener roller; F: Stripper roller; G: Spicked lattice; H: Delivery chute; I: Beater roller; J: Back oscillating sheet; K: Fulcrum of; L: Return roller.

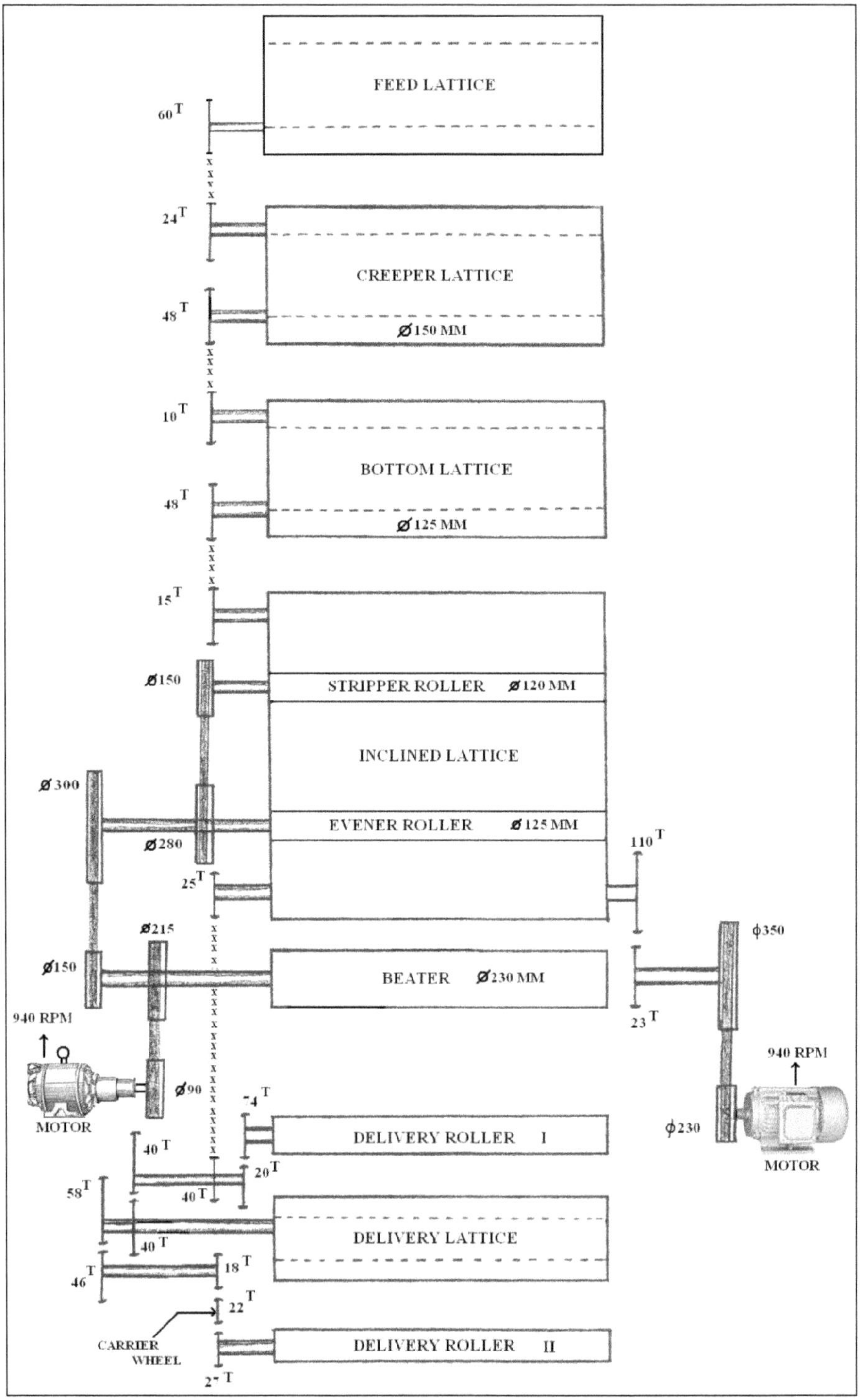

Figure 5.5: Hopper Feeder.

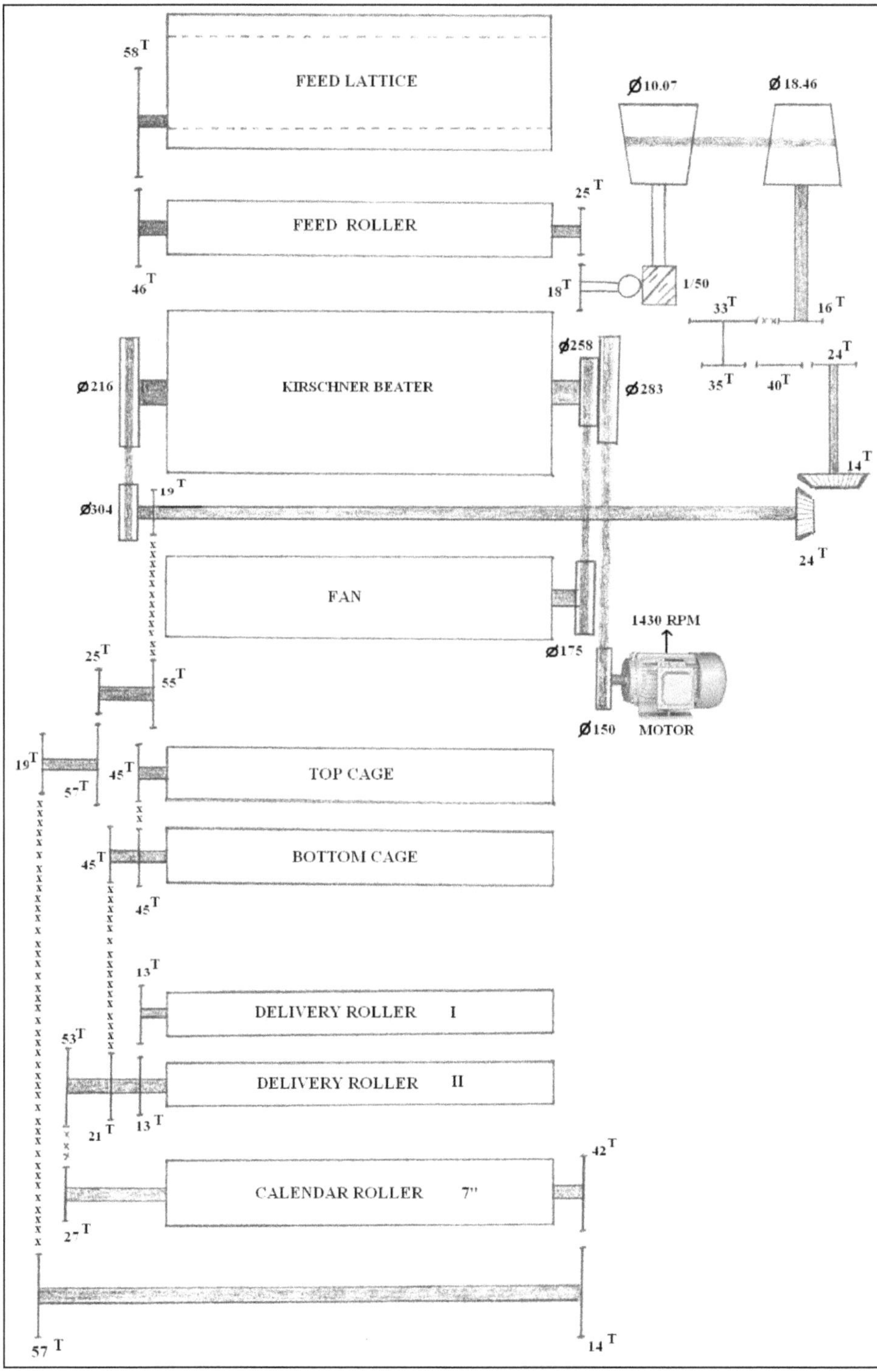

Figure 5.6: Kirschner Beater.

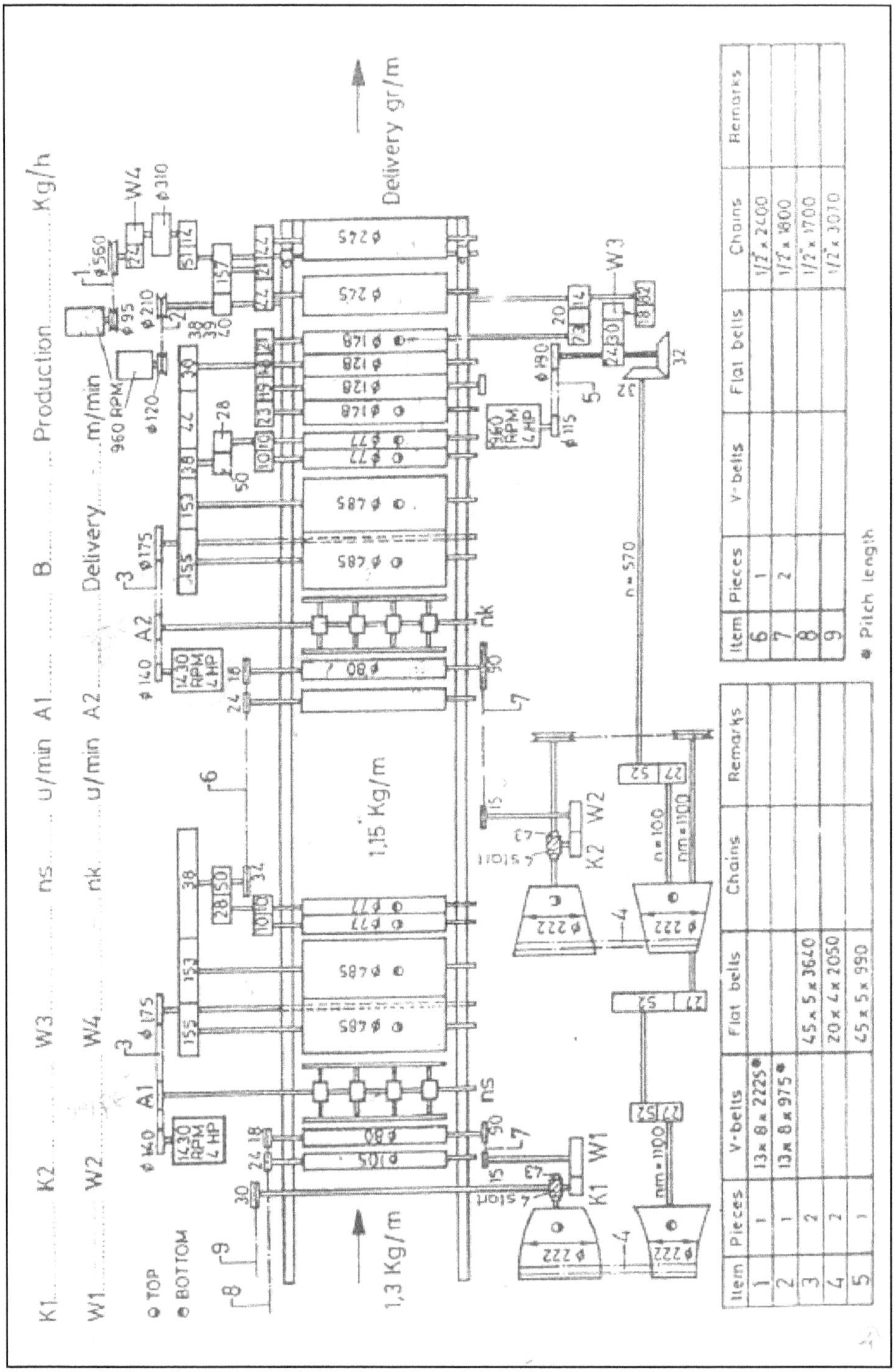

Figure 5.7: Scutcher Unit.

shaft D, on which mounted a large toothed wheel E, which in turn is geared into a small pinion F. This pinion is mounted on a short shaft, at one end of which is the hand wheel G, provided to permit the operative to release the pressure when doffing the lap.

At the other end of the short shaft is the brake drum H, against which a brake pad, fitted with suitable brake lining, is made to press by means of the weight J, which is adjustable. This weight is carried on lever K pivoted at L and with a high ratio of leverage exerts considerable upward pressure on lever M, which has its fulcrum at N and which carries the brake pad O. The forward end of the lever K has a suitable foot pedal P, which when depressed by the operative, releases the braking pressure on the drum H and so permits the operative to raise or lower the lap racks for doffing and restarting. It will be seen that, as the lap increases in diameter, the racks lift. So rotating the pinion F and transmitting motion through the gears to the drum G, this has to turn against the brake action, thus exerting a considerable pressure on the lap throughout the whole period of formation.

Measuring or Knock-Off Motion

An accurate measuring motion for the length of the lap is essential because the weight per yard of the lap is based on the total weight of the lap, on the assumption that the length of the lap is kept constant. If there is any small variation in yardage of the lap, it is reflected in total weight and weighing to determine the uniformity of the lap rendered valueless.

Limitations of Conventional Scutchers

1. The frequent use of conventional hopper feeders forms stringiness in fibres due to constant rolling of the fibres.
2. The sensitivity of mechanical regulator motion is affected due to inertia resulted in time lag.
3. The method of feeding to the intensive final beater by the roller and pedals is far from satisfactory.
4. Frequent stoppage of scutcher for lap doffing affects production and increases the workload of the operative.
5. Human error is involved in weighing and correction, which affects uniformity of laps.

4. PROCEDURE

1. Draw the complete gearing diagram of the machine
2. Show by arrow the flow of motion starting from motor to various parts
3. Mark various change pulleys / gears
4. Note down the diameters of the pulleys number of teeth of the gears and number of rows of spikes on evener roller.
5. List the various setting points.

5. CALCULATIONS

1. Calculate the rotational speeds of feed roller, beater, delivery roller, cages and fan in RPM and tabulate the results.

6. RESULTS

Tabulate the results.

	Feed Roller	*Beater*	*Delivery Roller*	*Cages*	*Fan Speed*
Rotational speed					
Surface speed					

6

Construction and Working Mechanism of HP Carding Machine

1. AIM

- ☆ To draw the motion transmission path from motor to various parts of the machine
- ☆ To observe the design features and important functional elements of the machine / mechanism
- ☆ To calculate the delivery rate in mpm, Individual draft, Total draft and Production of the machine in Kgs / Shift.
- ☆ To identify the change pulleys / gears.

2. FORMULA

Refer spinning useful formula relevant to your experiment

3. DESCRIPTION

The carding operation is the most important phase of short staple spinning. "Well carded is half spun" is an old expression that applies equally today. In the modern carding process there are three basic functions that have to be considered, namely:

- ☆ Lap formation using the chute feeding system
- ☆ The carding steps to produce a sliver and
- ☆ The control systems to facilitate the production of high quality sliver at increased production rates.

Carding Functions

The chute should supply a matt to the card which is uniform in mass and consistent in fibre openness

- ☆ The card opens the fibre tufts into individual fibres
- ☆ Removes a high proportion of the neps
- ☆ In the case of cotton, removes a majority of the trash
- ☆ Blends fibres in the short term
- ☆ Initiates fibre orientation
- ☆ Produces a continuous sliver of controlled mass.

TECHNOLOGICAL FUNCTIONS

The complex functions of the card will be described in detail in the following sections.

1. Opening the Fibre Tufts

Opening the fibre tufts into their individual fibres is the primary purpose of the card. As a result of the actions of the ginning process, the cleaning steps in the blowroom and the fans used to transport fibres between machines, entangled and knotted fibre bundles are created. These bundles are frequently referred to as – horseshoes, starfish, buttons, slubs and neps. If these bundles are not eliminated, the spinning process will be limited to coarse counts and the yarn quality will be low.

2. Elimination of Impurities

Elimination of foreign matter occurs mainly but not exclusively in the region of the licker-in. Only a small part of the contaminants is carried along with the flat strippings, or falls out at other positions. The degree of cleaning achieved by the modern card is very high, in the range of 80 - 95%. Thus, the overall degree of cleaning achieved by the blow room and the carding room together is as high as 95 - 99%. But carded sliver still contains 0.05 - 0.3% of foreign matter.

3. Elimination of Dust

In addition to free dust, which can be directly extracted by suction as in the blowroom, the card also removes a large proportion of the micro particles that are bound to the fibers. Significant fiber / metal or fiber / fiber friction is needed in order to loosen such particles. Both are available on the card to a considerable degree, *i.e.* the card is a good dust removing machine.

4. Disentangling Neps

While the number of neps increases from machine to machine in the blow room, the card reduces the remaining number to a small fraction. It is often falsely assumed that neps are eliminated at the card; in fact, they are mostly opened out. Only a fraction of the neps leaves the machine unopened via the flat strippings.

An improvement in the disentangling of neps is obtained by:

- ☆ Reducing fiber density on the cylinder by using larger cylinder widths;
- ☆ Closer spacing between the clothing surfaces;
- ☆ Sharper clothing;
- ☆ Optimal (not too low) licker-in speeds;
- ☆ Low doffer speeds;
- ☆ Lower throughput.

5. Elimination of Short Fibers

Short fibers can only be eliminated if they are pressed into and retained in the clothing. Since that is not possible with metallic clothing, only the flats can be considered in this context. The ability to select short as opposed to long fibers is based on the fact that long fibers have more contact with the clothing of the main cylinder than the short fibers. Thus longer fibers are continually caught and carried along by the main cylinder. Short fibers, on the other hand, offer fewer surfaces to the clothing of the main cylinder; they therefore remain caught in the flats clothing, are pressed into it and leave the machine in the flat strippings. Elimination of short fibers in the card must, however, be viewed in proportion. It is actually very small, as can be readily demonstrated. The card eliminates 1 - 2% flat strippings. Approximately half of the strippings are made up of short fibers. The card therefore eliminates fewer than 1% short fibers. In the staple diagram this is scarcely noticeable – the inaccuracy of the staple measurement procedure is greater than the change in value.

6. Fiber Blending

The card scarcely improves long-term blending, since the time spent by the material in the machine is too short. However, it improves transverse blending and fiber-to-fiber blending because, apart from the OE spinner, the card is the only machine to process individual fibers. Intimate fiber-to-fiber mixing is achieved in the formation of the web.

7. Fiber Orientation

Parallelizing action is often attributed to the card. This is not completely justified, since the fibers in the web are not parallel, although they do have, for the first time, a certain degree of longitudinal order. It is true that a parallel condition is achieved on the main cylinder, but it disappears during formation of the web between the cylinder and the doffer. Thus, the card can be given the task of creating partial longitudinal orientation of the fibers, but not that of creating parallelization.

8. Sliver Formation

In order to be able to deposit the fiber material, transport it and process it further, an appropriate intermediate product must be formed. This is the sliver. In extreme cases, card sliver has a count of 3 ktex (new spinning processes) to 9 ktex. Generally the count lies between 4 and 7 ktex (for direct feeding of drawframes up to 20 ktex) in the short-staple spinning mill.

OPERATING PRINCIPLE

In modern installations, raw material is supplied via pipe ducting into the feed chute (of different designs) (2) of the card. An evenly compressed batt of about 500 - 900 ktex is formed in the chute. A transport roller (3) forwards this batt to the feed arrangement (4). This consists of a feed roller and a feeder plate designed to push the sheet of fiber slowly into the operating range of the licker-in (5) while maintaining optimal clamping.

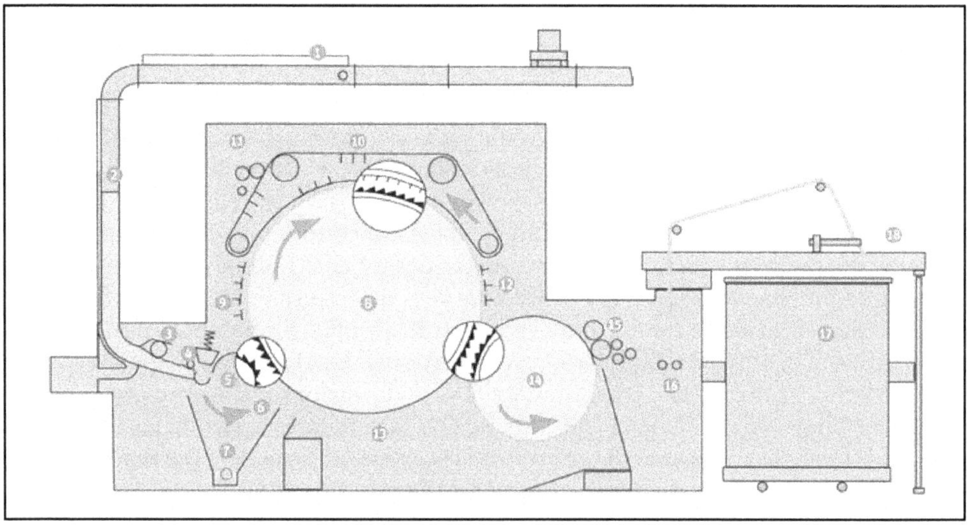

Figure 6.1: Modern High-Performance Card.

The portion of the sheet projecting from the feed roller must be combed through and opened into tufts by the licker-in. These tufts are passed over grid equipment (6) and transferred to the main cylinder (8). In moving past mote knives, grids, carding segments (6), etc., the material loses the majority of its impurities. Suction ducts (7) carry away the waste. The tufts themselves are carried along with the main cylinder and opened up into individual fibers between the cylinder and the flats in the actual carding process.

The flats (10) comprise 80 - 116 individual carding bars combined into a belt moving on an endless path. Nowadays some 30 - 46 (modern cards about 27) of the flats are located in the carding position relative to the main cylinder; the rest are on the return run. During this return, a cleaning unit (11) strips fibers, neps and foreign matter from the bars. Fixed carding bars (9) and (12) are designed to assist the operation of the card. Grids or cover plates (13) enclose the underside of the main cylinder. After the carding operation has been completed, the main cylinder carries along the fibers that are loose and lie parallel without hooks. However, in this condition the fibers do not form a transportable intermediate product. An additional cylinder, the doffer (14), is required for this purpose. The doffer combines the fibers into a web because of its substantially lower peripheral speed relative to the main cylinder.

CARDING ELEMENTS

1. Chute Feed System

In the blow room one or two fine opener / cleaners open the fibres and feed them into the distribution system. The fibres pass through the fan and are blown into the

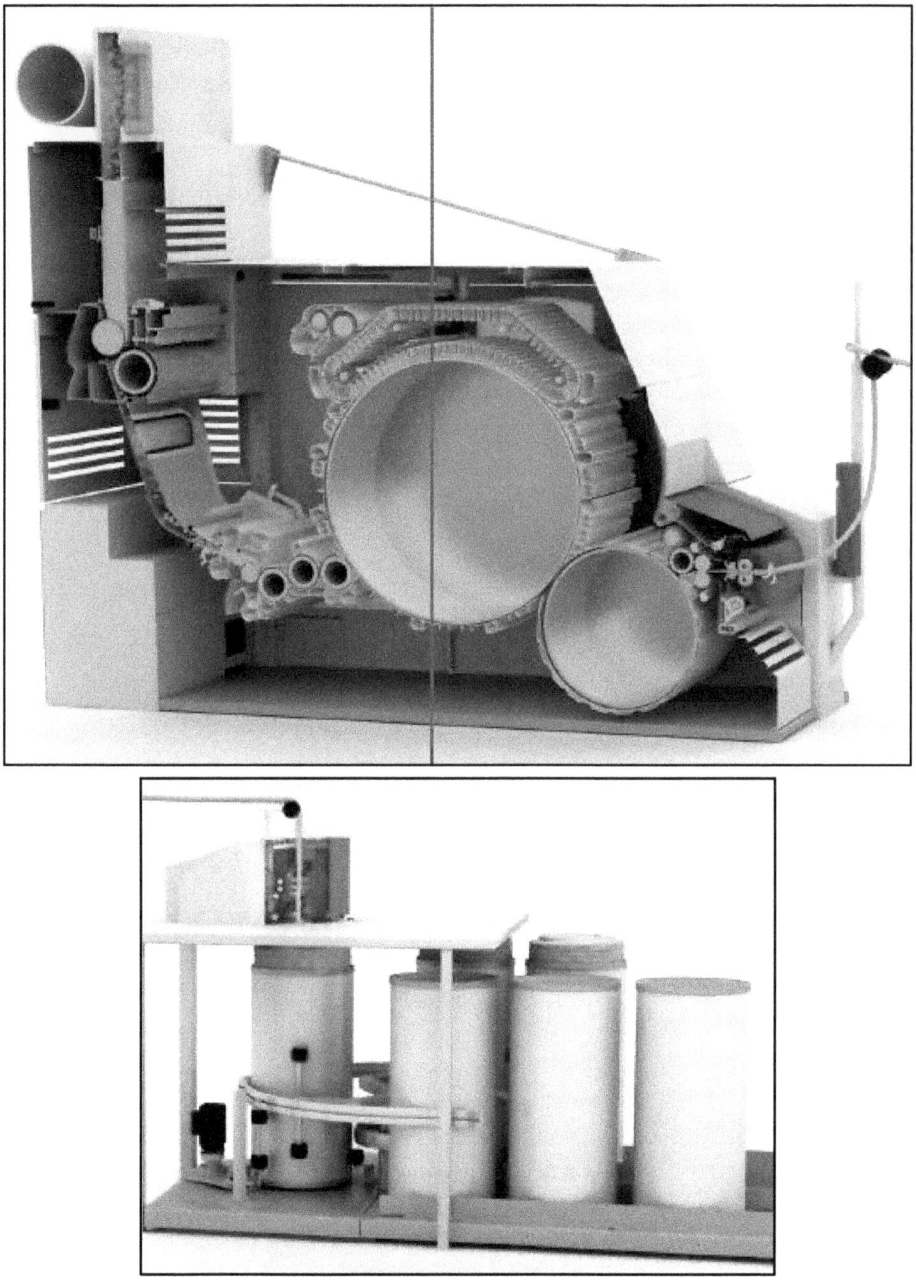

Figure 6.2: Trutzschler Card TC'06.

transportation ducts that pass over the tops of the chutes. The top chamber of the chute has a perforated side sheet though which the transporting air flows.

All of the transportation air has to pass through the perforated sheets, and depending upon the degree of chute filling the fibre passes to the chute with the least resistance to air flow. When all top chambers of the chutes are full, there is reduced airflow and the over-pressure increases in the feeding ducts. A pressure sensitive switch, between the fan and the first chute detects the pressure increase and stops the feeding machine. Similarly, when the air pressure drops to a pre-set low level the feeding machine is again started.

Function of the Integrated Chute

The chute is integrated into the card and thus is a vital component of the card for ensuring optimal overall operation of the card. The chute is part of the aerofeed pneumatic card feeding system. It can be used in a linear arrangement or in the "U" form. A cross-sectional view of a typical chute is shown in the illustration. The fan blows the fibres through the fibre duct (1). Gravity and the airflow cause the fibres to fill the upper feed chamber (2). The transport air passes through the perforated sheet into the extraction air duct. As fibre is fed to the lower chute, the perforated sheet is

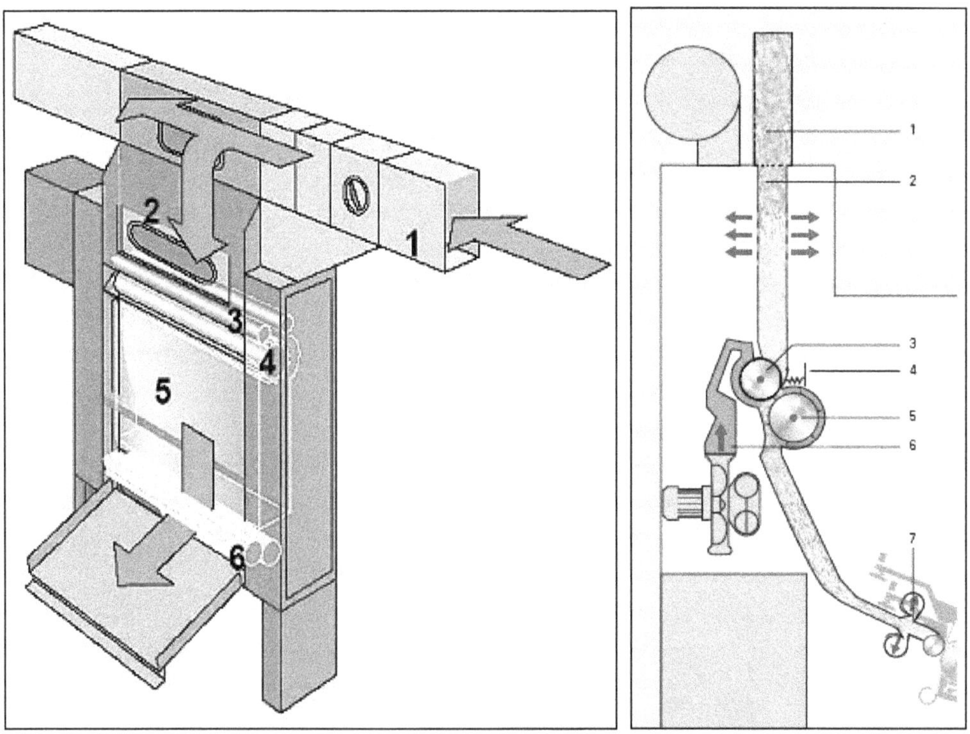

Figure 6.3: Tuft Feeder Directfeed.

1: High-volume upper trunk; 1: Integrtaed air volume separator; 3: Feed roll, electrically coupled to the card's feed roll; 4: Segmented tray for secure clamping; 5: Opening rolle with gentle needling; 6: Closed air circuit with integrated fan; 7: Self-cleaning air outlet combs.

exposed allowing more air to flow bringing additional fibre to the upper chute. The upper feeding chamber is equipped with a single feed roller (3), a feeding plate with a defined nipping point to control the fibre flow to the opening roller (4), which opens the material into tufts and transport the lower chute (5).

Fibre Batt Compression in the Chute

The standard version has a closed air circulation system, which is powered by a fan.

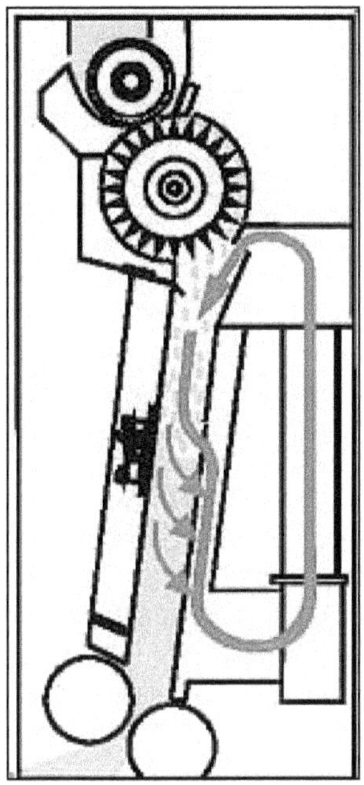

Figure 6.4: Chute Feed System.

The integrated fan controllers the air flow and effects even fibre compression across the width. A set of light scanning sensors monitors the material level in the lower chute and regulates the speed of the upper feed roller to maintain a controlled level and batt mass. The batt weight is primarily governed with the lower light sensor, which is in control during normal production speed.

The upper light scanner keeps the filling level slightly higher during the "creep speed" operation of the C 60 card. By adjusting the positions of the chute walls inward or out, the batt weight and volume can be influenced. The batt is taken from the bottom of the lower chute by the feed rollers (6) and fed to the card.

2. Feed and Licker-in

The unidirectional feed arrangement which transfers the fibres to the licker-in without a rapid change of direction which is the case with the convention feed roll/feed plate arrangement.

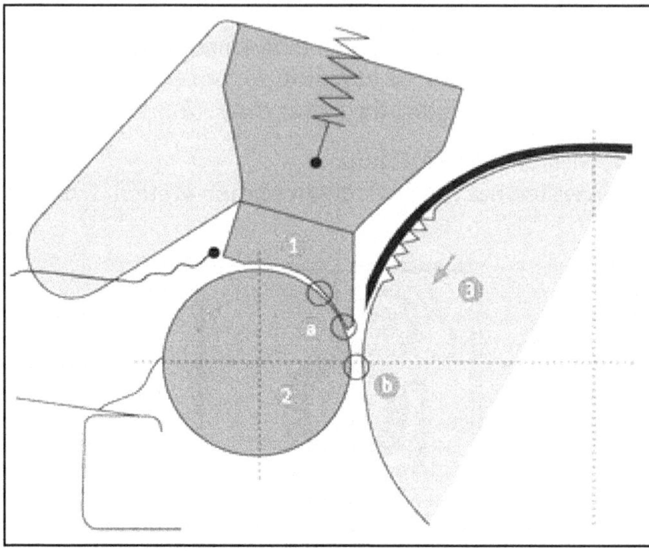

Figure 6.5: Uni-directional Feed.

The first tuft opening action takes place at the feeding point. The matt is firmly held between the feed plate and the feed roll and the licker-in separates fibres and tufts from the matt. The intensity of this action is dependent upon the speed of the licker-in and the setting of the feed plate. If the feed plate is set too close there will be fibre damage. As the fibres are fed, they are instantaneously accelerated to the surface speed of the licker-in, which is in the region of 900 m/min. (licker-in circumference x rpm. *i.e.* diameter – 250 mm x π x 1100 rpm = 864 m/min or 14.4 m/sec). If the matt feed rate were 1.6 m/min, the draft at the feeding zone would be 540:1

Licker-in Mote Knives and Carding Elements

The licker-in region is designed to remove trash and vegetable matter. Approximately 90% of the card waste is removed in the licker-in zone. This waste is high in trash content and is not re-usable. Preferably, it should not be mixed with the remainder of the card waste that is of higher fibre content and can be recycled for specific end uses.

The new licker-in assembly consists of adjustment free profiles with a new patented mounting. Two carding elements are fastened to each profile. With this innovation there is no need to adjust the carding element/licker-in distance. This reduces the assembly time when changing the licker-in and guarantees optimum running conditions.

3. Pre-carding and Post-carding Elements

As carding production rates have progressively been increased, it has become necessary to include additional stationary carding segments around the cylinder. They are located between the licker-in and the flats and between the flats and the doffer. In the first versions, the carding segments between the licker-in and the flats were used to progressively open up the tufts carried by the cylinder wire before the

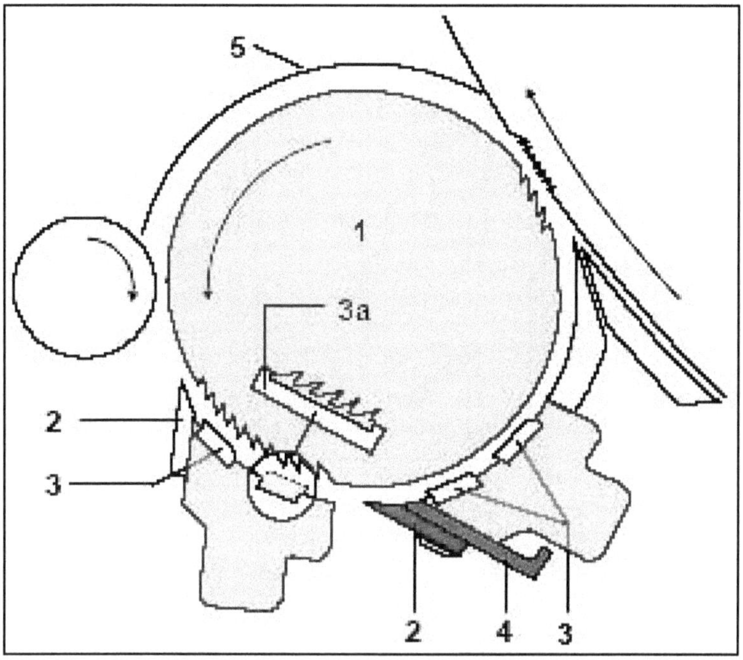

Figure 6.6: Licker-in Under Segment.

1: Licker-in; 2: Adjustable knife; 3: Carding element; 3a: Guide element; 4: Combi-profile.

fibres encountered the flats. Additionally, carding segments between the flats and the doffer were found to be beneficial in preparing the fibres for the doffing action. In the Rieter card these segments are referred to as the TREX-system. Developments of the carding elements and of suction channels located between the elements have led to TREXplus that removes dust, trash and very short fibres (Figure 6.7).

4. Flats

The primary carding action takes place between the cylinder and the flats. The fibres carried by the cylinder wire tend to move toward the flats that resist fibre movement. Many of the fibres "float" between the flats and the cylinder wire.

This "carding action":

- ☆ Separates individual fibres,
- ☆ Opens entangled fibres,
- ☆ Separates and retains the neps in the flats,
- ☆ Frees / removes trash particles and vegetable matter from the fibres,
- ☆ Removes dust collected in the flat strips,
- ☆ Orients the fibres in the direction of the cylinder movement.

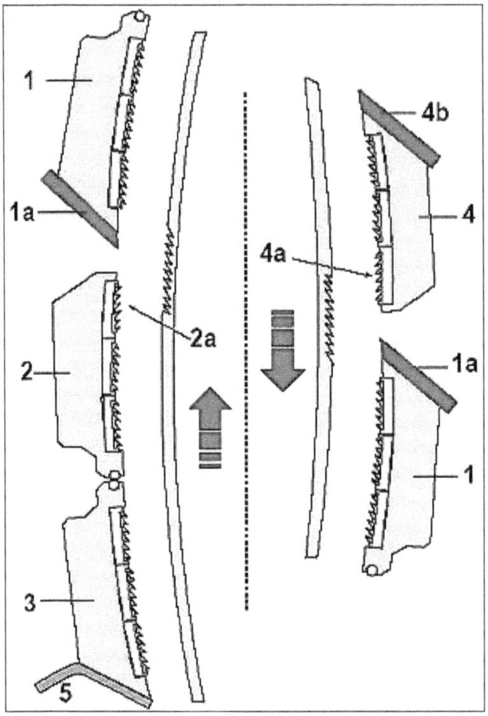

The TREXplus carding elements:

1 holder with a knife (1a) and 3 carding elements

2 holder the guide element (2a) and 2 carding elements

3 holder with 3 carding elements

4 holder with knife, guide element (4a) and 2 carding elements

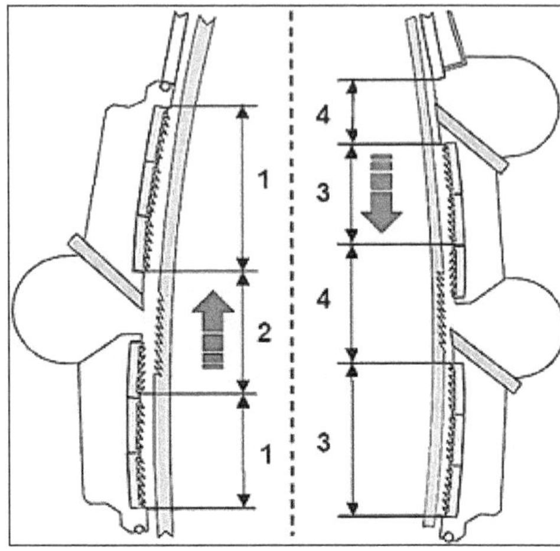

TREXplus selective trash removal:

Pre-carding zone,

1 Fibre opening,
2 Dust, trash and short fibre separation.

Post-carding zone,

3 Fibre opening,
4 Dust trash and short fibre separation.

The TREXplus system incorporates the toothed guiding elements that were developed to keep the good fibre on the cylinder wire while allowing the trash to ride on the surface and be removed at the trash slot.

Figure 6.7: Pre-carding and Post-carding Elements.

The carding surface of the flats is ground at a slight incline to allow the fibres to enter the space between the flats and cylinder. In conventional cards this means that the flat setting and closest distances between flat and cylinder is only at the trailing edge of the flats. Rieter uses a flat design with a "Heel" that increases the degree of carding at the trailing edge.

The setting of the flats is extremely important and has to be performed carefully according the instruction manual.

Direction of Flats Movement

The flats on Rieter's cards are moved backwards, that means the working flats move from the doffer side to the licker-in side. This is in the opposite direction of the cylinder movement.

The advantages of backward movement are:

- ✰ The first four or five flats over the licker-in take up the vast majority of the trash removed by the flats. This occurs regardless of the direction of movement of the flats.
- ✰ When the flats move in the backward direction, the trash taken up by the flats at the entry to the carding zone is immediately removed from the carding zone.
- ✰ The fibres passing through the carding zone move passed progressively cleaner flats as they approach the doffer. There is less tendency for impurities to be returned to the fibres on the cylinder because the last few flats are relatively clean.

5. Doffer

The fibres are removed from the cylinder by the "doffer". They rotate so that the cylinder and doffer surfaces move in the same direction at the transfer zone.

- ✰ The doffer rotates at a considerably slower surface speed than does the cylinder and consequently fibres accumulate on the doffer wire.
- ✰ The doffer speed is normally in range of 50 to 120 m / min and the cylinder surface speed is in the region of 1500 m / min.
- ✰ The doffer takes some of the fibres carried by the cylinder, but the majority stays on the cylinder. There is a transfer factor in the order of 0.2 to 0.3,
- ✰ Fibres, on average, pass around the cylinder 3 to 5 times.

The fibres taken up by the doffer are caught (hooked) on the wire and partially combed out by the passing cylinder wire. Consequently the fibres on the doffer have a majority of "trailing" hooks relative to the movement of the doffer and subsequent sliver. The fibres taken up by the doffer have to be held securely by the wire and must not drop from the wire as the doffer rotates.

The fibre transfer factor largely depends upon:

- ✰ the setting of the doffer to the cylinder,
- ✰ the type of doffer and cylinder clothing,
- ✰ the wire tooth geometry, particularly of the doffer,
- ✰ the number of points on the cylinder and doffer,
- ✰ the sharpness of the doffer wire,
- ✰ the aerodynamics at the exit region of the cylinder doffer zone.

6. Cylinder Plates and Tongue

The tongue is located between the doffer and cylinder underneath the doffing zone. It is used to minimize air disturbance and facilitate a smooth and consistent transfer of fibre to the doffer. The tongue is pre set and normally does not need to be adjusted. On the other hand, for certain carding conditions, re-setting may be necessary or even a modified tongue may be needed.

Under the cylinder Rieter installs cylinder cover plates that do not allow waste to be discharged. In high speed carding the quality is better when solid plates are used and the air turbulence under the card is eliminated.

7. Sliver Formation

The web on the doffer is removed by a detaching roller that has to be set to peel off the web in a smooth continuous action. The setting distance between the detaching roller and the doffer depends upon the web weight and the bulkiness of the fibres being carded. A "protective plate" is provided under the detaching roller to prevent the peeled web from breaking or dropping from the detaching roller. The web is then taken up by the top and bottom delivery rollers, there being a transfer roller nestled between the detaching roller and the delivery rollers to ensure a smooth web movement.

The web emerging from the delivery rollers is gathered by the traversing cross apron that carries the fibre assembly to the sliver-forming zone. The material first passes through a "condensing" trumpet and is then pulled through the compacting trumpet by the stepped rollers. From the stepped rollers the sliver is transported to the coiler. The relative speeds of the elements of the delivery section have to be adjusted according to the delivery speed and the nature of the material being processed. The respective drafts should be set according to the instruction manual.

8. Sliver Coiling

There are two types of coilers available:

- ✰ The rotating can coiler in which the coiler plate deposits the sliver coils into a can that is revolving.
- ✰ The planetary coiler in which the can is stationary and the coiler plate is moved to lay the coils and form the sliver column.

In either system the setting of the coiler has to be done to prevent sliver damage, stretching, or over filling the can. The sliver column should be 8 to 10 mm clear of the can sides to allow easy withdrawal of the sliver at the Drawframe.

9. Sliver Count Auto Levelling

The card sliver usually presents some variations in count (long-term irregularities) due mainly to the section of entry lap. Less frequently, sectional irregularities on short lengths of sliver are generated (the so-called short-term irregularities). These are eliminated by the doubling of slivers on the drawframe.

A device called a self-regulator is used to highlight the variations in count on the card. By varying the drawing action of the machine on the basis of the variations in the section of material, the device permits slivers to be obtained with maximum evenness.

The autoleveller is composed of:

- ✰ A measuring device which controls, on entry or on delivery, the section of fibrous mass being worked and sends signals with proportional intensity to the measured section;

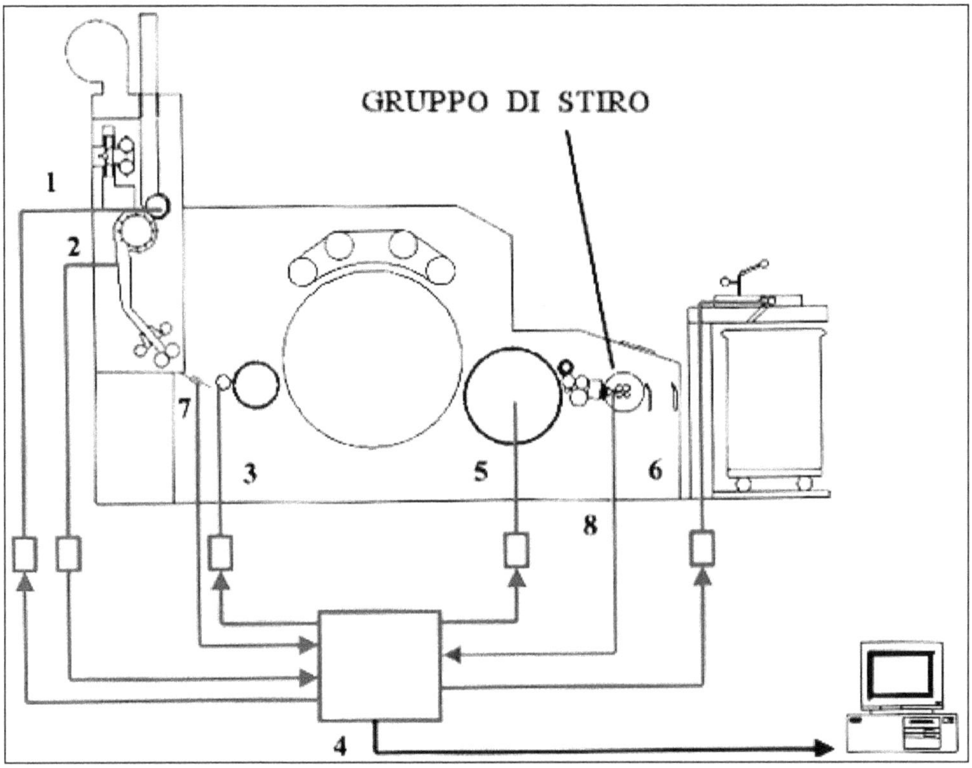

Figure 6.8: Auto Levelling in Card.

1: Hopper feeder cylinder; 2: Analogue pressure switch; 3: Card feeder cylinder; 4: Microcomputer; 5: Doffer; 6: Coiler; 7: Lap thickness sensor; 8: Funnel with monitoring sensor for quantity of sliver.

- ✰ An electronic apparatus that processes and recognizes the data sent by the measuring device and, if the difference between the measured value and the desired value is greater than the preset tolerance level, it sends electrical impulses to the draft variator;
- ✰ A speed variator controlling the movement of the autoleveller, that carries out the variation of the machine draft on the basis of the section of material controlled.

Depending on the position of the measuring and levelling devices, there are closed loop auto levellers when the measuring device is placed before the autoleveller or on open loop autoleveller when the contrary occurs.

4. PROCEDURE

1. Draw the complete gearing diagram of the machine
2. Show by arrow the flow of motion starting from motor to various parts
3. Mark various change pulleys / gears

4. Note down the diameters of the pulleys number of teeth of the gears
5. List the various setting points.

5. CALCULATIONS

1. Calculate speeds, surface speeds of the various organs.
2. Calculate the speed ratios in order to find out drafts
3. Plot a graph showing change in draft as a function of draft change pinion.

6. RESULTS

Tabulate the results.

	Lap Roller	*Feed Roller Roller*	*Taker-in*	*Cylinder*	*Doffer*	*Flats*	*Calendar Roller*	*Coiler Calendar*
Rotational speed (rpm)								
Surface speed								

Part of Card	*Surface Speed Ratio or Draft*	*Draft Constant of the Machine*
Lap roller : Feed roller		
Feed roller : Taker-in		
Taker-in : Cylinder		
Cylinder : Doffer		
Doffer : Calendar roller		
Calendar roller : Coiler cal. Roller		
TOTAL		

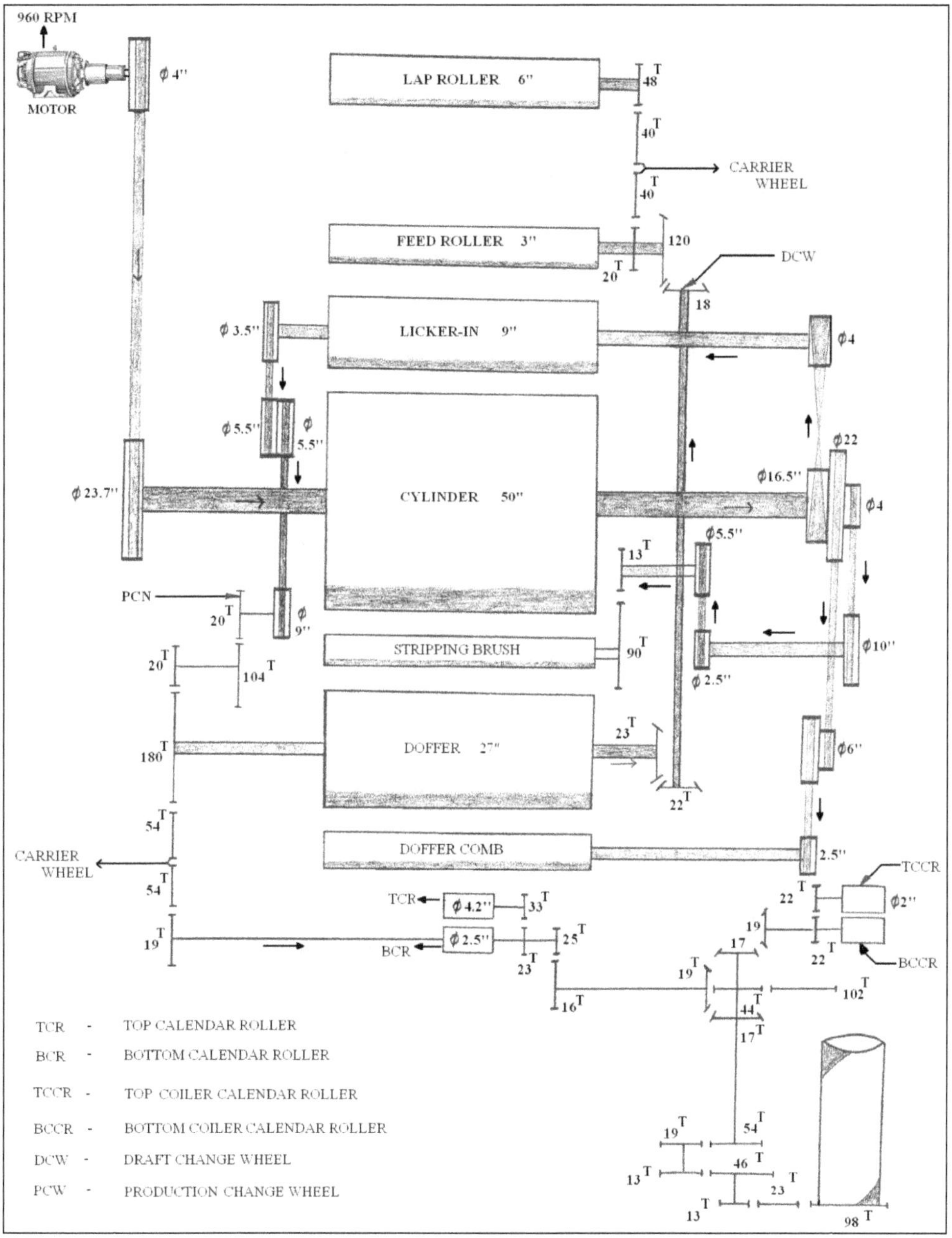

Figure 6.9: Carding Machine.

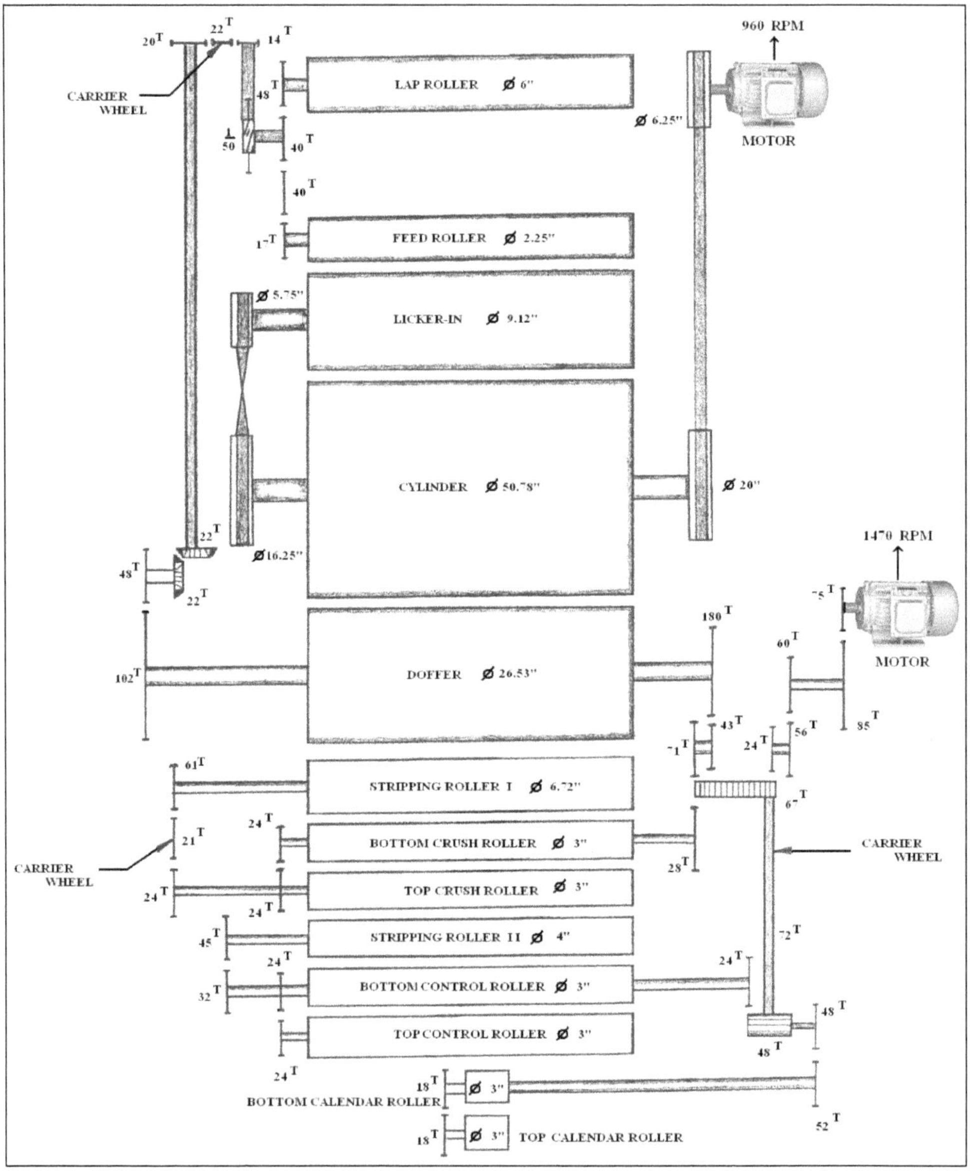

Figure 6.10: High Speed Carding Machine.

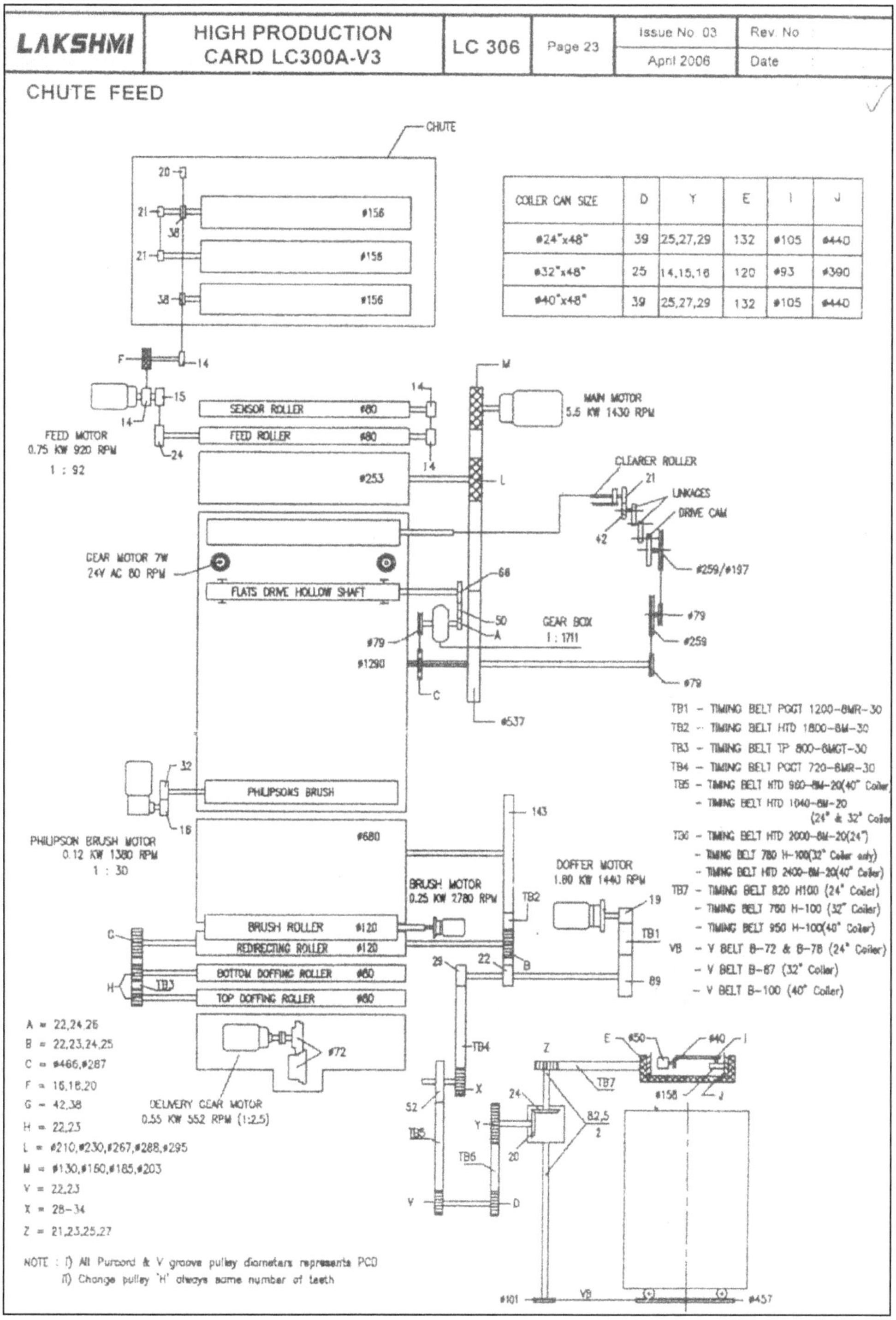

Figure 6.11: LMW Carding Machine–Chute Feed.

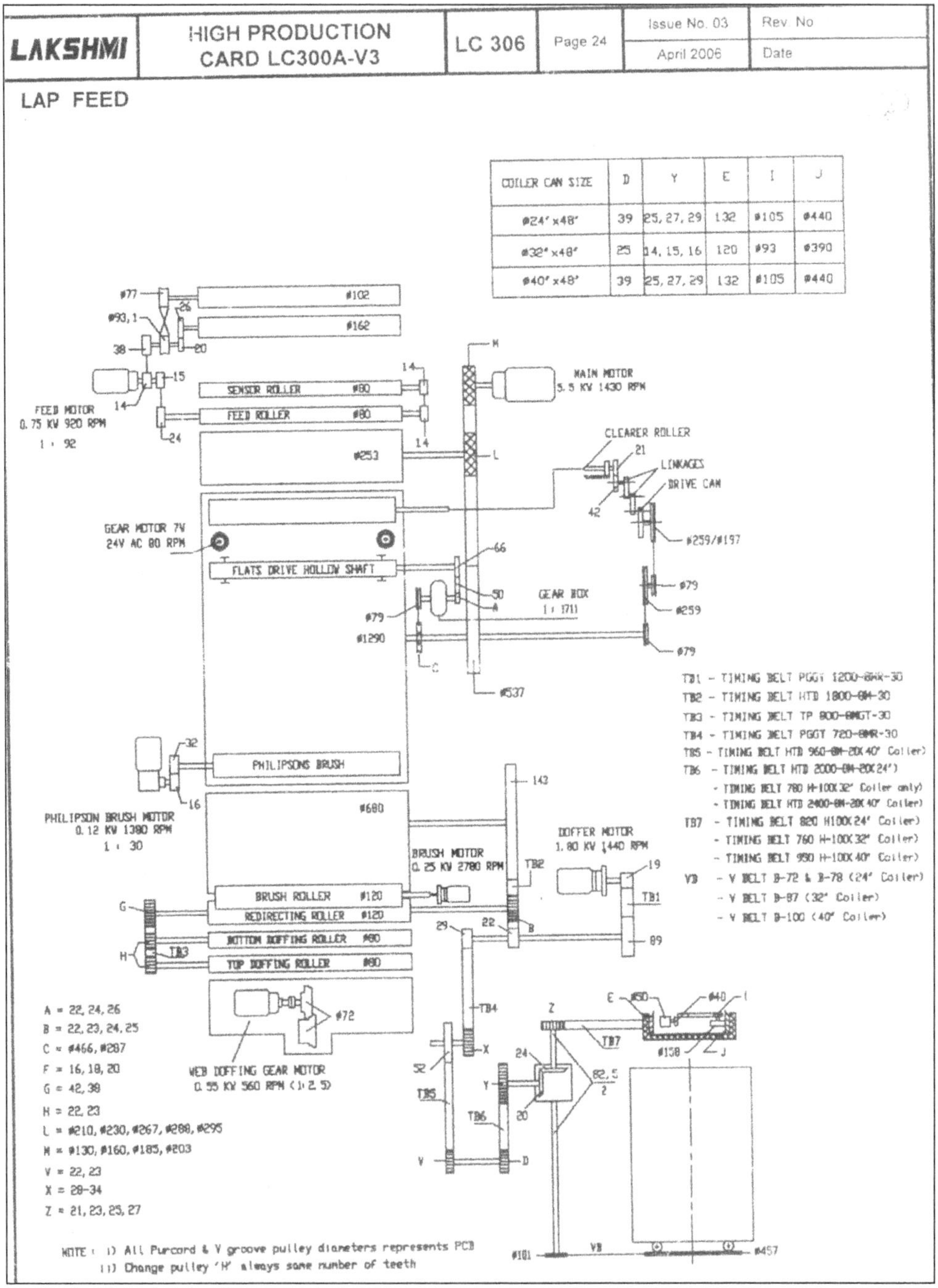

Figure 6.12: LMW Carding Machine–Lap Feed.

7

Study of Various Setting Points in Carding Machine and their Effect on Sliver and Yarn Quality

1. AIM

- ✰ To draw the setting diagram of the machine
- ✰ To study the setting points for processing cotton and synthetic fibres
- ✰ To study the influence of setting points on yarn quality.

2. FORMULA

Refer spinning useful formula relevant to your experiment

3. DESCRIPTION

SETTING POINTS IN CARDING

1. Matt Weight and Condition

- ✰ The best matt weight is when the carding draft is in the optimal range. For most fibres a carding draft of 95 to 125 is targeted.
- ✰ It is important that the matt should be consistent from side to side. Lengthwise variation can be corrected by the levelling system but irregularities across the matt cannot be accommodated. Holes or thin places in the matt are problematic because the fibres are not fully controlled at the feeding zone.

- ☆ Matt draft should not be too low with buckled matt feed. Nor should it be so high as to pull thin places. Drafts are available from 1.19 to1.37.
- ☆ A test for buckling is to remove tufts of fibre from the matt as it is being fed and see if the matt tends to lift with the tufts. If it does lift, increase the tension.
- ☆ A more consistent matt is produced when the chute feeding system is running at a high production ratio. It should be running for more than 90 percent of the time for best results.
- ☆ The material should be well opened with no compacted or entangled material.

2. Feed Plate Setting

The adjustment of the feed plate (feed trough) is normally made according to the fibre staple length. The recommendation from the manual can be used as an approximate guideline:

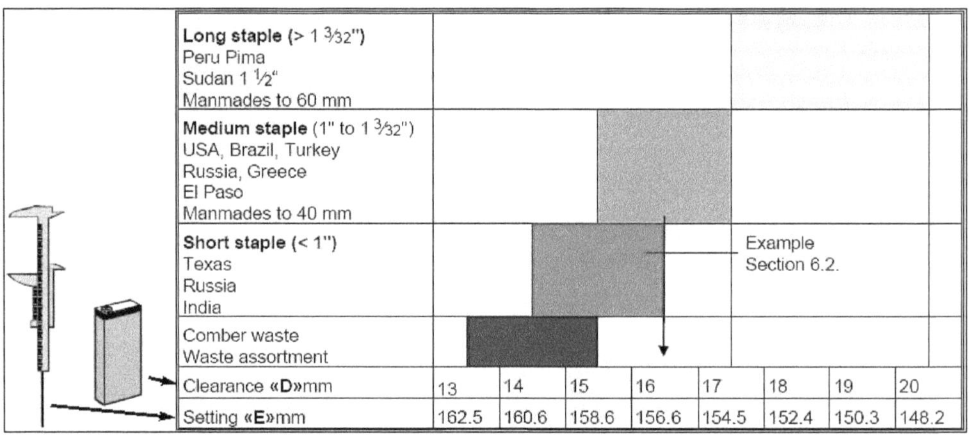

Figure 7.1: Adjustment of Feed Trough.

Determination of Nipping Point "D"/Carding Point.

Care should be taken to see that fibres are not being over controlled at the feeding point. If the longest fibres are being broken, the feed plate setting should be opened up.

3. Licker-in and Cylinder Speeds Ranges by Fibre Types

The following table shows the C 51 Hi•Per•Card typical speed ranges for man-made fibres, cotton and trashy cotton. This information should be used in conjunction with the charts below referring to production rates.

	Licher-in Speed (rpm)	*Cyliner Speed (rpm)*
Synthetics and blends	900 to 1300	300 to 450
Cotton	1610 to 2160	450 to 600
Trashy cotton	1000 to 2000	300 to 600

4. Licker-in/Cylinder Fibre Transfer

The material on the licker-in is transferred to the cylinder. At the transfer zone the licker-in wire is in the doffing position relative to the cylinder, which has a higher surface speed. The cylinder is travelling in the same direction as the licker-in and therefore the opening effect is small.

Generally, the ratio of licker-in surface speed to cylinder surface speed should be about 1:2. Changing the licker in speed to maximize trash removal alters this ratio. Care should be taken to ensure that increasing the licker-in speed to remove more trash does not compromise the overall carding performance. The licker-in speed is linked to the cylinder speed but there are three ratio changes that can be made and the recommendations are:

Man-made fibres and bleds	Cylinder/licker-in ratio 2.05 ("slow" licker-in speed)
Cotton	Cylinder/licker-in ratio 1.78 ("medium" licker-in speed)
Cotton with a high trash content	Cylinder/licker-in ratio 1.55 ("fast " licker-in speed and standard for the C51 Hi•Per•Card)

Immediately after the cylinder takes the fibres they are pressed into the wire by the cylinder cover plate. The plate has to be set relative to the cylinder wire to ensure that the wire securely transports the fibres.

5. Licker-in Segment Settings

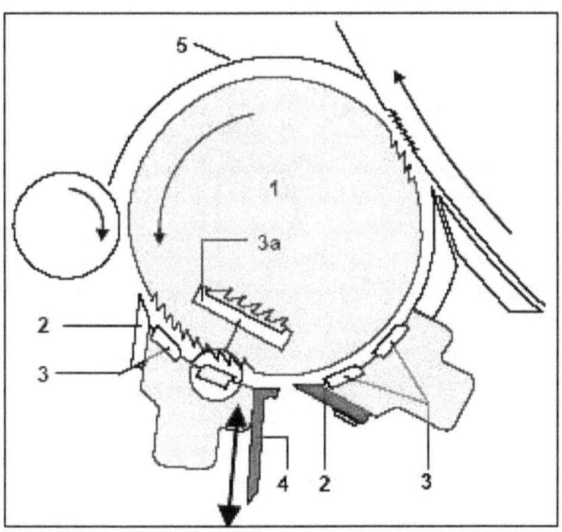

Figure 7.2: For Cotton

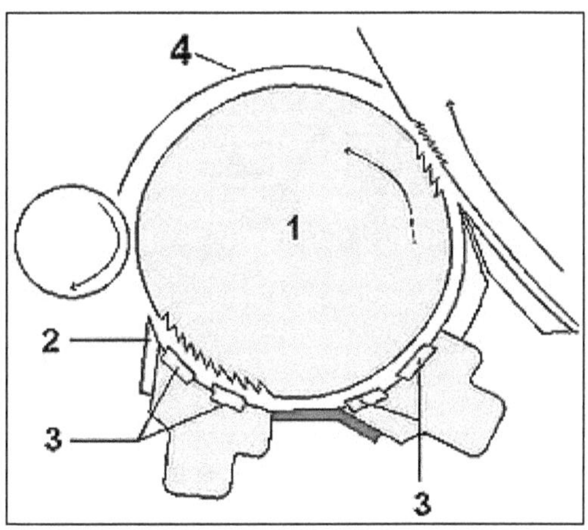

Figure 7.3: For Synthetic fibres

In the above illustrations of the C51 Hi•Per•Card, there are two knives and two profiles shown in each case. It is also normal to use a single knife and one profile when carding short clean fibres such as cotton noil. Additionally, for man-made fibres it is possible to use a single profile with either a single knife or a "feeding aid" can be used to replace the knife and eliminate waste being removed at the licker-in.

The degree of waste removal and cleaning at the licker-in is influenced by:

- ☆ The setting of the knife relative to the licker-in wire,
- ☆ The size of the trash removal opening immediately before the knife,
- ☆ The number of knives,
- ☆ Speed of the licker-in: higher speeds increase waste removal, but may also increase fibre damage,
- ☆ With heavier matt weights the feeding speed is lower and the fibre is held for a longer time in the opening zone. This increases the opening action of the licker-in and slightly increases the trash removal but there is also a tendency to damage fibres.

BASIC SETTINGS AROUND THE CYLINDER

The standard values for settings around the cylinder are included in the machine manual. A typical example from the C 51 manual is shown in Figure 7.4. Doffer/ Cylinder Settings for Cotton and Blends

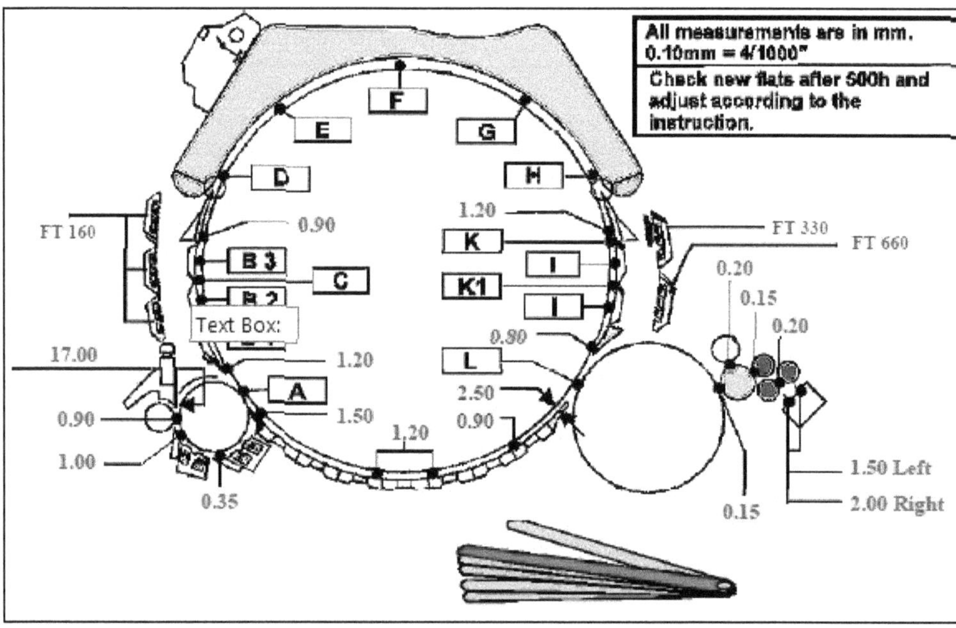

Figure 7.4: Setting Points in a Carding Machine.

In the constant effort to maximize nep and trash removal there is a tendency for the customer to request closer settings of the flats, segments and doffer relative to the cylinder. Great care has to be given to very close settings, with attention being given to:

- ☆ Setting when the card is warm or cold,
- ☆ Cylinder speed, if the speed is increased the warm running settings become closer,

- ☆ The condition of the clothing on the flats, cylinder and doffer. It may be prudent to "dress the clothing before closing up on the settings.
- ☆ If flats are changed or new clothing installed it is necessary to dress the flats before adjusting to tight settings.
- ☆ After re-clothing the card, it should be "run –in" before going to high speed and close settings.

Doffer

The following chart is taken from the C 51 Hi•Per•Card manual and shows the basic cold machine settings of the doffer to the cylinder for a production range of 50 to 90 kg/hr.

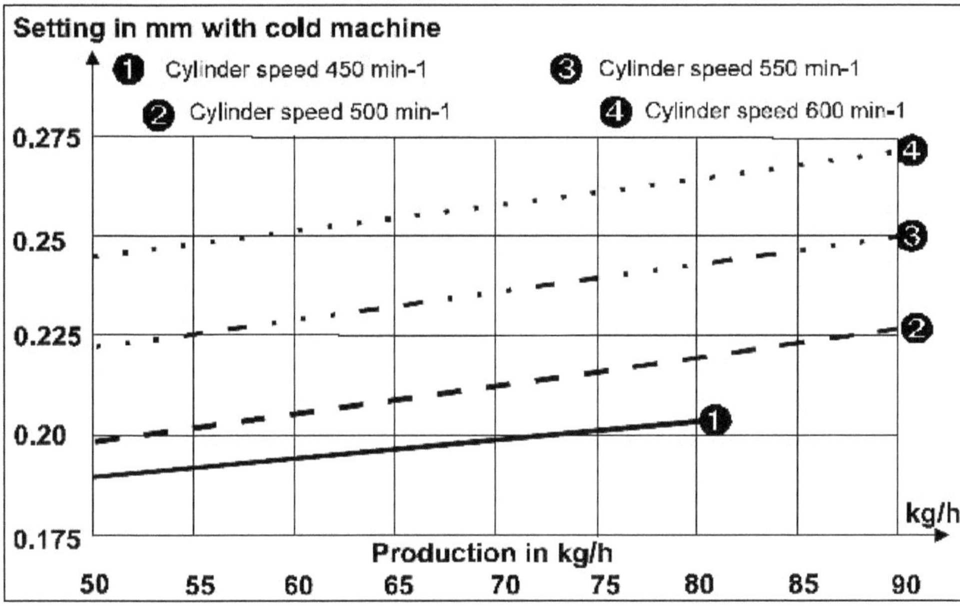

Figure 7.5: Setting between Cylinder and Doffer.

Carding Synthetic Fibres

Processing synthetic fibres on high-production cards requires "high performance fibre finish" to adequately lubricate the fibre and provide satisfactory antistatic properties. Heat is generated by the carding action and is transmitted to the card clothing. Overheated clothing encourages static charging of the fibres, making it difficult to detach the web.

Increasing the moisture content of the surrounding air by increasing the humidity can reduce electrostatic charging of the fibres. However, this should not include increasing the room temperature. Try to keep the fibres from overheating.

When the synthetic fibres are well opened in the blowroom it is easier to process them at the card. With well-prepared fibres it is possible to operate the cards with wider flat settings, hence the friction forces and static charging are minimized.

The effectiveness of the fibre finish varies. In most cases it is at its best between two to three weeks after the date of manufacture, after which it deteriorates steadily. It is preferable to have the fibre delivered as needed and not to store bales for several months.

The rate of finish degradation varies from one supplier to another and in many instances from batch to batch from the same supplier. Consequently, changing from one batch to another should be phased in over several days.

Fibre Crimp

The crimp of synthetic fibres affects the production rate of the card. Strong fibre crimp gives the card web better cohesion and web stability. To set a strong fibre crimp, the fibre producers use higher pressures and temperatures in the fibre production process. The additional heat treatment usually means a loss of fibre strength that is translated into a loss of yarn strength. Consequently, these high crimp fibres are not used in high strength applications such as sewing threads. To card low crimp fibres the production rates have to be reduced and sometimes the card web weight has to be increased.

IMPACT OF MACHINE SETTINGS

The complex function of the card requires that the settings and conditions of the elements be correct. The following are a few examples of what can happen when the settings are incorrect:

1. Feed Roller to Licker-in
   - ☆ Setting too close:

     Loss in yarn strength and elongation

     Fibre damage, increased short fibre content.
   - ☆ Setting too wide:

     Thick places in the yarn, (increased CV%)

     Insufficient trash removal.
2. Feed Trough (Plate) Nipping Distance (D)
   - ☆ Setting too close:

     Fibre damage

     Loss in yarn breaking strength
   - ☆ Setting too wide:

     Thick places in the yarn, (increased CV%)

     Insufficient trash removal.
3. Licker-in to Cylinder
   - ☆ Setting too close:

     Possible fibre damage

     Danger of early cylinder wire damage.

☆ Setting too open:

Possibly excessive flat strips.

4. Flats to Cylinder

☆ Settings too close:

Loading of the cylinder

Static accumulation

Damage to flats and cylinder wire

☆ Settings too wide:

High nep count in the sliver

Insufficient fibre orientation

Insufficient trash removal

5. Cylinder to Doffer

☆ Settings too close:

Damage to the cylinder and doffer wire, "Facing"

☆ Settings too wide:

Loading of the cylinder

Uncontrolled fibre transfer

High nep count in the sliver

Cloudy web.

6. Tongue to Cylinder and Doffer

Tongue to close: - Fibre collects on the tongue and causes the web to break. Tongue should be lowered to increase the distance from the nip and swung to obtain a clean fibre transfer.

Tongue too open: - For waste and short fibres the tongue may have to be set closer to obtain clean fibre transfer.

REASONS FOR SLIVER BREAKS

Trash Accumulations at the Condenser

☆ Obviously worse with dirty cotton. The card has to be cleaned frequently to prevent trash build-up.

☆ Excessive short fibres cause accumulations. - Check fibre in the laydown and waste handling procedures as well as possible card related reasons.

☆ When the doffer wire is not sharp the short fibres and fly become "airborne" and contaminate the delivery system.

☆ Any doffer wire that does not hold the fibre web creates fly under the doffer and dust in the take-off area.

Irregular Fibre Transfer between Doffer and Stepped Rollers

☆ Check the draft settings of the transfer rolls to ensure sooth web transfer. If necessary revert to the basic settings and adjust until the web is "quiet".

Bad Doffer Condition

- ☆ Check the draft settings of the transfer rolls to ensure sooth web transfer. If necessary revert to the basic settings and adjust until the web is "quiet".
- ☆ As mentioned above when the wire is not sharp the fly is increased,
- ☆ The doffer wire can be contaminated with trash particles embedded in the wire. If this is so, it is necessary to manually brush the doffer until it is clean.
- ☆ If the wire is loaded with fibre finish due to some "off quality" fibre, try to brush it clean. If this does not work, it may be possible to process some coarse easy to run fibre that will clean the wire by running.

REASONS FOR HIGHER NEPS IN CARD SLIVER

Nep Removal Efficiency (NRE) in card can be expressed in percentage and calculated as

$$\text{NRE}\,\% = \frac{(\text{Neps/Gm in Feed - Neps/Gm in Delivery}) \times 100}{\text{Neps / Gm in Feed}}$$

Contribution from Machinery Parameter

Parameter	*Influence%*
Type of Card Clothing Wire	20%
Wire Sharpness of Card clothing	40%
Flat to Flat Height variation and Flat to Cylinder Setting	50%
SFD Setting	10%
Cylinder RPM	15%
Waste Percentage	20%
Relative Humidity	20%
Productivity	Directly related with increase in production

Contribution from Material Parameter

Parameter	*Influence*
Micronaire	Lower the micronaire, higher Neps in sliver
Type of trash in the mixing	Higher low weight trash like leaf bits, higher Neps in sliver
Maturity of Cotton	Lower the maturity level, higher Sliver Neps

Parameter	*Influence*
Neps in Feed material	Nep Generation is high with rupture in BR will lead to Higher Neps
Honey Dew Content	Higher Honey Content, Higher Neps in sliver

Control of Neps in Card

For reduction of neps in carding we have to consider the following factors:

1. Wire sharpness of card clothing
2. Flat to flat height variation
3. Flat to Cylinder setting
4. Cylinder speed
5. SFD setting
6. Relative Humidity
7. Waste percentage and
8. Production (doffer speed and sliver hank)

1. Wire Sharpness of Card Clothing

The guideline for wire population and speeds for producing quality sliver are given below:

Fibres	Very fine Yarn combed Ring	Med-Fine Yarn combed Nm 100	Coarse Yarn Carded / OE	Man Made > 1.0 dtex – 3.3	Man Made < 1.0 dtex – 0.6
Yarn count	> Nm 80 (>Ne 48)	Nm 40 .... 100 (Ne 24 .... 60)	< Nm 35 (< Ne 20)		
Licker-in					
- PPSI	41	41–61	41–61	32	36 pin roller
- angle	10 deg.	10 deg.	10 to 15 deg.	0 to 5 deg.	58 deg.
- rpm	900–1300	1000–1450	1300–1700	800–1100	1430
Cylinder					
- PPSI	800–1080	800 to 1000	600–865	450 to 650	720
- angle	30 deg.	40 deg.	30 deg.	30 deg.	30 deg.
- rpm	350–450	400–500	450- 600	400–450	400–450
Flat clothing	550	480	410	350	430
Doffer					
- PPSI	340–365	340–365	280–340	280–340	340–365
- angle	30 deg.	30 deg.	30 deg.	30 deg.	30 deg.

The primary indication that the clothing needs to be ground is that the nep count in the sliver has reached the upper tolerable limit. The wire condition should be visually checked using a magnifying glass of 30 to 50 powers. The tips of worn clothing appear rounded with no carding leading edge. It is then necessary to grind the clothing until a clean sharp leading edge is visible over the whole of the clothing.

The recommended grinding interval and life of the different card clothings are given as a guideline:

	Life (Tones)	*1st Sharpening*	*2nd Sharpening*	*3rd Sharpening*	*4th Sharpening*	*5th Sharpening*
Cylinder wire	450	No Sharpening is needed. If the Flat Tops are changed at 350 tones, the wire may give life up to 700 tones				
Flat tops	400	100	180	260	340	Replace

For Sharpening the Flat Tops, Full width Emery Roller to be used. Once in alternate Grinding, Full width Ceramic stone is used for leveling. For synthetic Tops, there is no sharpening needed

Licker-in wire	120 to 150	No sharpening for Licker-in. Life depends on Trash level / fibre stickiness in Cotton
SFD	450	No sharpening for SFD.
SFL	120 to 150	No Sharpening for SFL
Doffer	450	Sharpening is need based or once in 100 Tones.

The grinding should be performed carefully and in small steps to prevent the formation of "burrs on the front edge of the teeth.

2. Flat to Flat Height Variation/Flat to Cylinder Setting

To increase the nep removal efficiency in card, the flat wire height variation should be minimum to ensure uniform setting between flat to cylinder at all points. Flat Height Variation to be measured with reference to cylinder. If it is measured in a jig, toe area to be measured

- ✰ Within Flat Variation 0.02mm
- ✰ Flat to Flat Variation +/- 0.02mm

Overall Range of Variation can be max of 0.05mm.

The factors influencing the Flat Height Variation are:

a) Method of Flat Clipping and Leveling - To get a perfect clipping, Flat to be clipped only after pasting. After loading the new flat, it is better to go for one ON machine flat leveling.

b) Off machine Wire Sharpening is not recommended.

c) Resting of Heel and Toe on Flexible bend to be ensured. If the flats are lifted up, the chain may be reason. Proper lubricating of the Chain and proper torque tightening of Flat bolts to be ensured.

d) Twist in the flat, which has to be corrected during re-clipping.

e) Wear out of Heel and toe Area - New Clipping to be done only after end Milling if the wear out is noticed.

f) Fibre Accumulation in the Flat Guide pulleys will tilt the flats.

3. Cylinder RPM

With higher Cylinder speed, slight reduction in the Neps/Gm and Nep Size can be noticed. However, in the process, the following negative impact on quality of sliver, which we need to be observed and corrected.

1) Increase in Waste%
2) Increase in SFC (n)%.

With the lower cylinder speed (Say 360RPM), the AFIS results may be good with respect to Neps/Gm and SFC(n), but yarn quality results may not be good. This is due to less opening at Carding due to lesser Cylinder RPM. Hence Optimum fibre opening must be ensured at Card. Other than DCH, No cotton will give quality results with 360Cylinder RPM.

4. SFD Setting

With the closer post carding segment settings, the NRE can be increased slightly due to better opening and cleaning action of already well opened fibres from the flat zone. For low production less than 20Kgs, 0.225 mm setting and for Higher Production above 20kgs, 0.25mm setting can be kept for better performance.

5. Relative Humidity

Relative humidity in the department plays an important role in nep reduction. Higher the RH in the department, lower the NRE and higher Neps/Gm in card sliver due to lack of opening and sticking of fibres in the machine parts. For Cotton like PIMA, the Temperature must be 100 to 103 F and RH% must be 42 to 45%. Normal Recommendation of RH% in carding department is 50 – 55%

6. Waste Percentage

Removal of higher waste in carding results in lower the Neps/Gm up to some point of waste level. Flat strips are the main waste which is responsible for nep removal which can be increased either by closer flat setting or by increasing the flat speed. Beyond certain limit, Neps/Gm will not come down as the waste percentage increases. It is better to take more waste in Comber than in card to have better quality

7. Productivity

Productivity and neps in card sliver are directly related *i.e.* as the productivity (depends on doffer speed and sliver hank) increases, the neps/gm in sliver will also increase due to lack of fibre opening and individualization in the flat region as the fibres will soon transferred to the doffer. The guidelines for the productivity level in card for better performance are given below:

- ☆ Up to 20's Count – Up to 55 Kgs/Hr
- ☆ 30's – 40 to 50 Kgs/Hr
- ☆ 40's – 30 to 40 Kgs/Hr
- ☆ 60's and above – Depending on Mixing and Quality requirement

HIGHER SLIVER TRASH%

If the trash removal rate is too low, check and correct the following.

- ☆ Check/correct the condition of the clothing on the:
  Licker-in,
  TREX elements,
  Cylinder.
- ☆ Check/correct the settings of:
  Knives on the licker-in, especially the first knife,
  Knives of the TREX,
  Flats to the cylinder, - standard settings are recommended
- ☆ Check/optimize the speeds of:
  Licker-in, - select the speed ratio corresponding to the type of cotton.
  Cylinder, - the speed should be consistent with the production rate.
- ☆ Check the influence of increasing the speed of the flats. If positive, inform plant personnel.
- ☆ Check/correct the waste suction system. Be sure that there are no chokes or bad connections.

HIGHER SHORT FIBRE CONTENT SLIVER

To minimize the SFC:

- ☆ Set the feed plate according to the staple length,
- ☆ New wire or clothing is aggressive and damages fibres. Speeds should be reduced during the running – in period.
- ☆ If the matt contains entangled fibres and lumps the SFC is increased. Check the characteristics of the matt and fibre in the blowroom.
- ☆ Ensure that the TREX settings are correct.
- ☆ Check to see that the card clothing is correctly specified and installed.
- ☆ Check the flat settings. If the flats are set too close to the cylinder, fibre damage can occur.
- ☆ Increasing the flat speed will increase the removal of the short fibre, but there is also an increase in overall flat strips.

IMPROVING THE SLIVER UNIFORMITY

The main influences of sliver uniformity are:

- ✰ The condition of the matt,
- ✰ The flat settings,
- ✰ The condition and settings of the doffer,
- ✰ The performance of the delivery section, doffer to the stepped rolls,
- ✰ Incorrect or insufficient blending,
- ✰ Variations in the amount of added reworkable waste.

Even though the card is equipped with an autoleveller it cannot make corrections for the small holes or lumps in the matt. Neither can it make a correction for any variation created within the card or the delivery section. Those irregularities that show up in the spectrogram can be addressed by identifying the defective component and making the necessary correction.

To otherwise improve the sliver uniformity it is necessary to visually identify the causes and then make the required adjustments.

4. PROCEDURE

Dismantle the carding machine up to Licker-in region and using leaf gauge the following settings should be done.

5. RESULTS

Sl.No.	*Setting Points*	*Cotton*	*Synthetics*
1.	Feed plate to licker-in		
2.	Feed roller to Feed plate		
3.	Licker-in under segments:		
	Combing segment I		
	Mote knife I		
	Combing segment II		
	Mote knife II		
	Licker-in grid		
4.	Licker-in to Cylinder		
5.	Back plate bottom		
6.	Back Plate Top		
7.	SFL:		
	SFL Bottom		
	Knife - ISFL Middle		
	Knife - IISFL top		

Sl.No.	*Setting Points*	*Cotton*	*Synthetics*
8.	Cylinder Under-casing:		
	Back		
	Front		
	Tongue height and Gap		
9.	Cylinder to Flats (5 points)		
10.	Front plate Top		
11.	Front Plate Bottom		
12.	SFD:		
	SFD -1		
	Knife		
13.	Cylinder to Doffer		
14.	Doffer to Re-directing roller		
15	RD Roller to Top crushing roller		
16	Top to Bottom crushing roller		

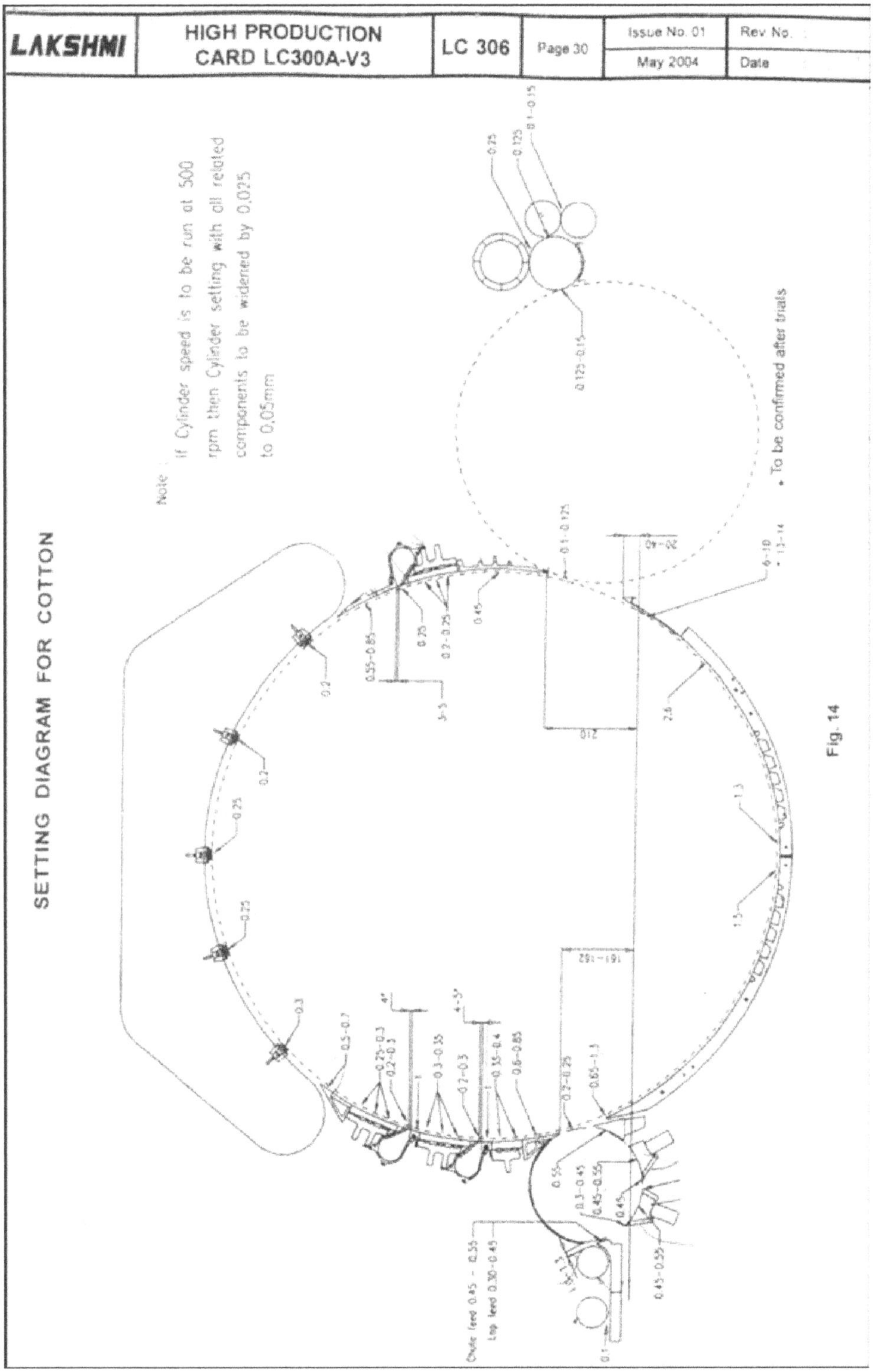

Figure 7.6: Setting Points for Cotton.

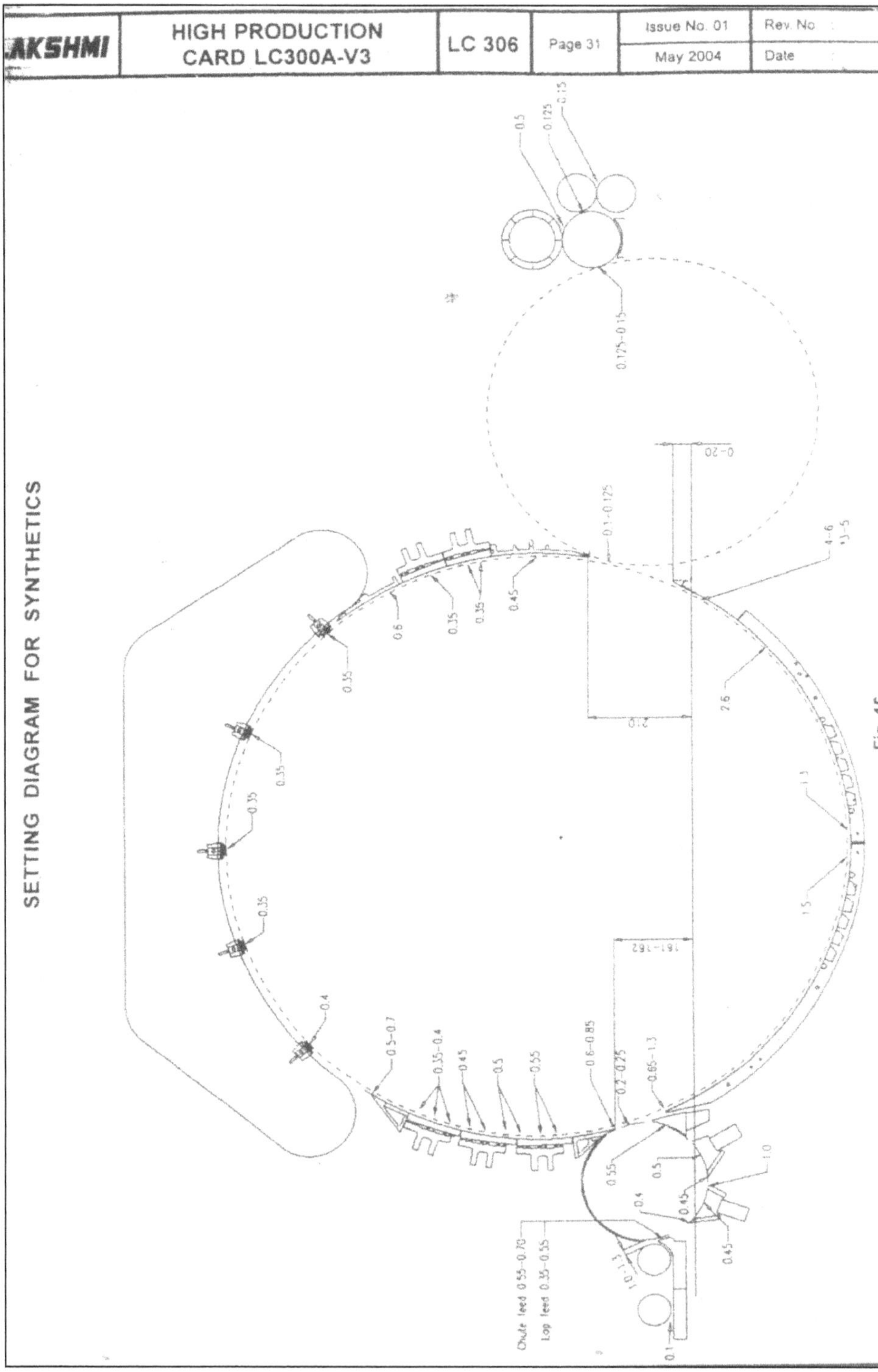

Figure 7.7: Setting Points for Synthetics.

8

Study of Card Wire Clothing and their Effect on Sliver and Yarn Quality

1. AIM

- ☆ To study the types of wire clothing
- ☆ To study the various specification in wire clothing
- ☆ To study the selection of wire clothing for Cotton and Synthetics.
- ☆ To compare the wire clothing of specifications and recommendations of different manufacturers

2. FORMULA

Refer spinning useful formula relevant to your experiment

3. DESCRIPTION

CHOICE OF CLOTHING

Of all the individual components of the card, the clothing has the greatest influence on quality and productivity. The development of new clothing enabled, for example, the production rate of the card to be increased from 5 kg/h to the current level of up to 220 kg/h. New clothing was not, of course, the only factor involved in this increase, but it made a major contribution to it. Unfortunately, a price has to be paid for this development in the form of a steadily increasing departure from any possibility of universal clothing, which was formerly aimed at. Mills now have to make a difficult choice between hundreds of available clothing types, a choice of the utmost importance. Selection criteria are:

- ✰ Type and design of card;
- ✰ Rotation speed of the cylinder;
- ✰ Production rate;
- ✰ Material throughput;
- ✰ Raw material type (natural or man-made fibers);
- ✰ Fiber characteristics (mainly fineness, length, bulk, dirt content);
- ✰ Overall quality requirements;
- ✰ Price of the clothing;
- ✰ Service offered by the clothing supplier.

Classification

If we consider not only the short-staple spinning mill, but all fields in which card clothing is used, thousands of variations are currently on offer. They can be divided into three groups.

1. Flexible Clothing

This features hooks of round or oval wire set into elastic, multiply cloth backing. Each hook is bent into a U-shape and is formed with a knee that flexes under bending load and returns to its original position when the load is removed. In short-staple spinning mills this clothing is now found, if at all, only on the card flats.

The substrate is formed as a continuous narrow band (51 mm for the main cylinder) or as a broad band (equal to the length of the flats) comprising five (flexible clothing), seven (semi-rigid clothing) or even more plies of cloth joined together by vulcanizing. Double hooks of round or oval wire are embedded in the substrate; each has a knee in the leg and a cross-bar at the foot. The knee is required so that the hook does not project too far outward when the leg is bent back; it is thus possible to operate with small spacings between the clothing surfaces. In order to make the clothing more aggressive, the points are mostly ground on both sides (lateral sharpening), and they are also hardened. In the flats, the point density is in the range of 240 - 500 points per square inch.

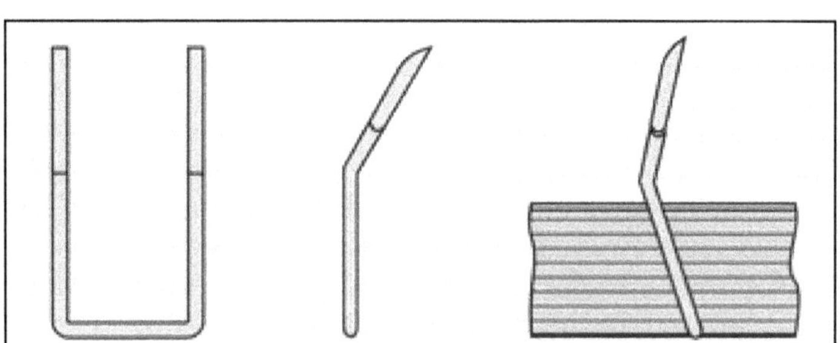

Figure 8.1: Flexible Clothing.

2. Semi-Rigid Clothing

In this, wires with square or round cross-sections and sharp points are set in backing which is less elastic than that of flexible clothing. This backing is a multi-ply structure with more plies than the backing of flexible clothing, comprising layers of both cloth and plastics. Flat wires are not formed with a knee, but round wires may have one. The wires cannot bend and are set so deeply in layers of cloth, and possibly foamed material, that they are practically immovable. When subjected to bending loads, they are therefore much less capable of yielding than flexible clothing types. They are also found only on the flats.

This clothing is similar in structure to the flexible types. However, it has more cloth layers (possibly also foamed material) and has hooks of wire with squared cross-sections without a knee, or of reinforced round wire with or without a knee. Compared with flexible clothing, it has the advantage that it does not choke with fiber and thus eliminate less flat strippings. In addition, it does not need sharpening as often as flexible clothing types. At least in respect to flat wires, it should be mentioned that each sharpening removes material from the tip so that the working surface becomes steadily broader and the aggressiveness of the clothing declines over time. This wire clothing without lateral sharpening can be re-sharpened only once or twice; with lateral sharpening up to four times.

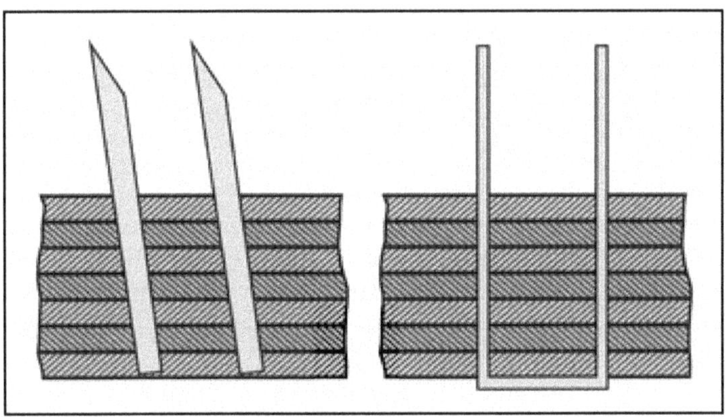

Figure 8.2: Semi-Rigid Clothing.

3. Metallic Clothing

These are continuous, self-supporting, square wire structures in which teeth are cut at the smallest possible spacings by a process resembling a punching operation. If the teeth are relatively large, for example as in the licker-in, the clothing is referred to as saw-tooth clothing. (The terms saw-tooth clothing and metallic clothing refer to the same thing.) Nowadays, the licker-in, main cylinder and doffer use metallic clothing without exception.

Manufacture of Metallic Clothing

The starting material is round wire, which is rolled in several stages to give the desired profile. This profiled stock is passed through a cutting machine. Here, a high-precision cutting tool, corresponding exactly to the shape of the gap between two teeth, punches (cuts) the wire away piece by piece between the teeth, which remain after the cutting operation. It is of the utmost importance that the dimensions are held within the finest tolerance limits. Hardening immediately follows cutting, *i.e.* the wire is passed through a flame and a quenching bath. Here also a high degree of uniformity is required, this time in the hardness achieved. The required 'feel' for this operation can only be appreciated when it is realized that in fine clothing the tip of the tooth has a thickness of only 0.05 - 0.06 mm.

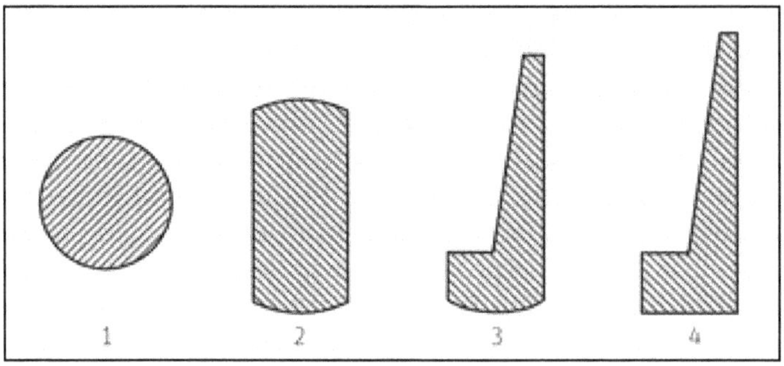

Figure 8.3: Forming the Wire Profile for Metallic Clothing.

Geometry of Card Clothing

Card wires are manufactured with a variety of rib-base designs depending on the application and machine concept. Some of the designs include surface wound, camlock and groove installation. Some of the technical descriptions and wire angles are as follows:

1. The shoulder thickness is the width of the rib or camlock and determines the distance from tooth-row to tooth-row. This influences the number of points per square inch and contributes to the strength of the surface area.

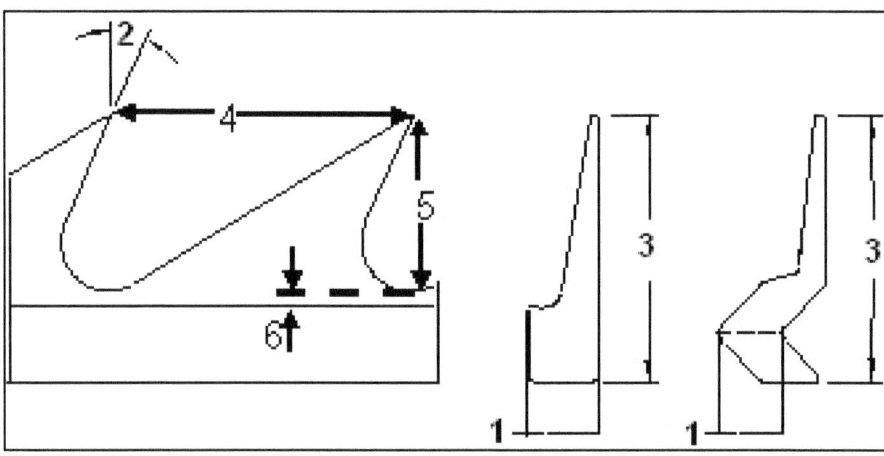

Figure 8.4: Wire Geometry.

1: Shoulder thickness; 2: Front angle; 3: Total height; 4: Pitch; 5: Height of tooth; 6: Web height.

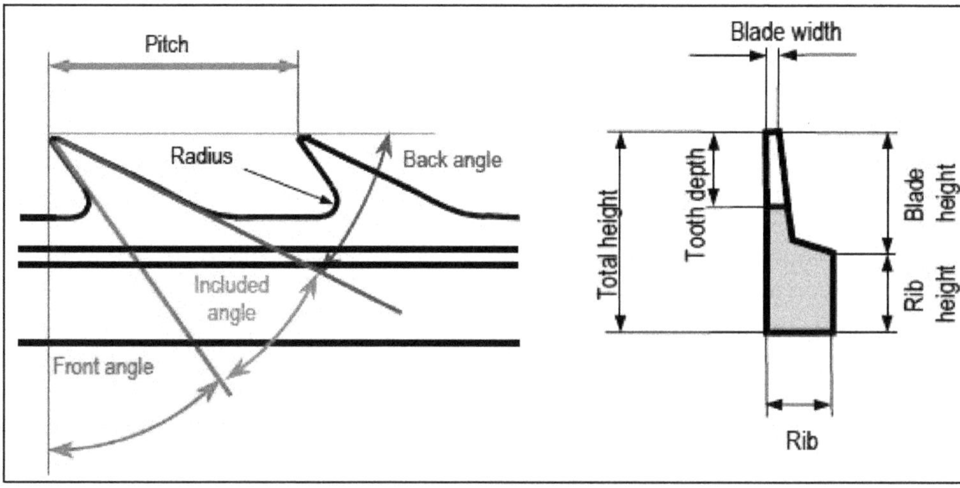

Figure 8.5: Wire Cross-Section.

2. The front angle is the fibre-carding angle, which is the main influence factor in the aggressiveness of the carding action. This angle limits the number of teeth per linear inch and placed demands on the cylinder speed. In addition, it determans the fiber holding capacity of the wire.
3. The total height of the wire contributes to the amount of fibres carried by the wire. It also contributes to the outer diameter of the clothed carding element.
4. The pitch is the distance from the tip of one tooth to the next. This determines the number of linear teeth per inch, the smaller the pitch the more teeth per linear distance.
5. The height of the cut tooth defines the capacity of the maximum fibers carried. On the cylinder application, the tooth height defines also the remaining web and fiber crossblending factor within the card.
6. The web height is the amount of the tooth left above the rib, which is not puched out. Trash particals can build up in this space, but air currents can also aid in the lift of fibers from the cylinder.
   - ☆ The back angle will affect the tooth strength. It will aid or hinder the release of the fibres from the wire.
   - ☆ The included angle is the result between the front and back angle and is the measurement of the tooth shape. The sum of the front, back and included angles is always 90 degrees.
   - ☆ The tooth side angle is the tilt from the tooth-point to the shoulder and defines the strength of the tooth. This wedge can aid or reduce the amount of trash build-up; cotton plant particles tend to be speared.
   - ☆ Point thickness. The sharper the point, the better the separation of fibres, but the easier it can be damaged. The wire must be rolled, punched, hardened and wound onto a reel without being damaged.
   - ☆ The radius contributes to the release of the fibres and the life of the wire.

The Most Important Operating Parameters of the Clothing

1. Point Density (Number of points per unit surface area)

The point (or tip) density has a significant influence on the carding operation. However, the number of points and the speed of rotation of the cylinder must be considered together. It is not simply the total number that is significant, but also the number available per unit of time, *i.e.* the product of the point density and the speed of movement of the surface. Thus, low point populations can be partially compensated by higher cylinder speeds. (This is not always possible, since the overall result may be deterioration in some quality parameters.)

It must also be kept in mind that the populations of the main cylinder and doffer clothing have to be adapted to each other. In general, the higher the point population, the better the carding effect – up to a certain optimum. Above that optimum, the positive influence becomes a negative one. This optimum is very dependent upon the material. Coarse fibers need fewer points, as they need more space in the card clothing; finer fibers must be processed with more points, since more fibers are present if the material throughput is the same. Point density is specified in terms of points per square inch or per square centimeter, and can be calculated as follows:

1. $$\text{Points Per Square Inch} = \frac{645}{\text{Base width (mm)} \times \text{Pitch (mm)}}$$

2. $$\text{Points Per Square Centimeter} = \frac{100}{\text{Base width (mm)} \times \text{Pitch (mm)}}$$

3. $$\text{Points Per Square Centimeter} = \frac{\text{Points Per Square Inch}}{6.45}$$

2. Base Width (a1)

This influences the point density. The narrower the base, the greater the number of turns that can be wound on the cylinder and, correspondingly, the higher the point population.

3. Height of the Clothing (h1)

The height of metallic clothing on the cylinder today varies between 2 mm and 3.8 mm. The height must be very uniform. It can also exert an influence on the population, since shorter teeth – for a given tooth carding angle – leave space for more teeth. Where shorter teeth are used, the fibers are less able to escape into the clothing during carding and better carding over the total surface is obtained. Clothing with smaller teeth is also less inclined to choke with dirt particles.

4. Tooth Pitch (T)

The population is also determined by the tip-to-tip spacing.

5. Carding Angle ($\propto$)

This is the most important angle of the tooth:

- ✰ The aggressiveness of the clothing; and
- ✰ The hold on the fibers are determined by this parameter.

The angle specifies the inclination of the leading face of the tooth to the vertical. It is described as positive (a,), negative (b) or neutral. The angle is neutral if the leading edge of the tooth lies in the vertical (0°). Clothing with negative angles is used only in the licker-in, when processing some man-made fibers.

Since the fibers are held less firmly by this form of tooth, they are transferred more easily to the cylinder and the clothing is less inclined to choke. Carding angles normally fall into the following ranges:

Licker-in	+5° to -10°
Cylinder	+12° to +27°
Doffer	+20° to +40°

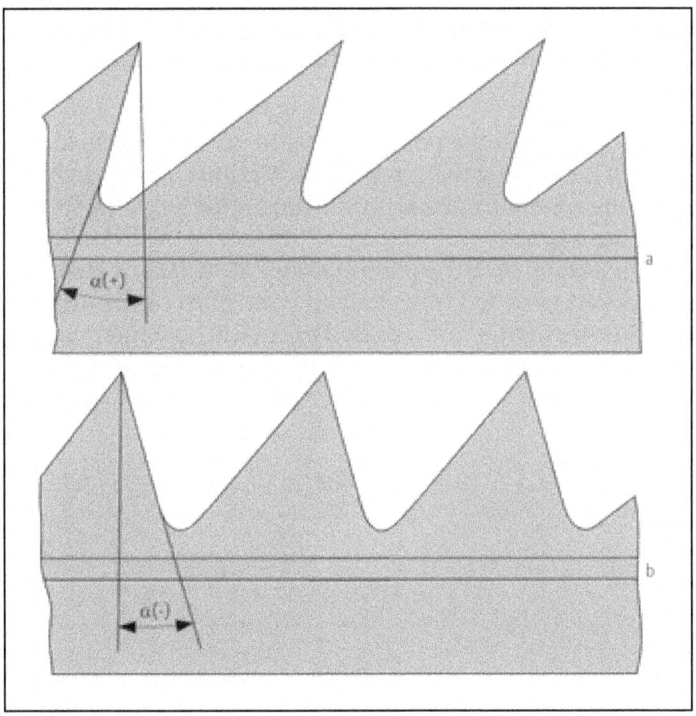

Figure 8.6: Positive (a) and Negative (b) Carding Angle.

6. The Tooth Point

Carding is performed at the tips of the teeth and the formation of the point is therefore important. For optimum operating conditions the point should have a surface or land (b) at its upper end rather than a needle form. This land should be as small as possible. To provide retaining power, the land should terminate in a sharp edge (a) at the front. Unfortunately, during processing of material this edge becomes steadily more rounded; the tooth point must therefore be re-sharpened from time to time. Formation of a burr at the edge (a) must be avoided during re-sharpening. The tooth

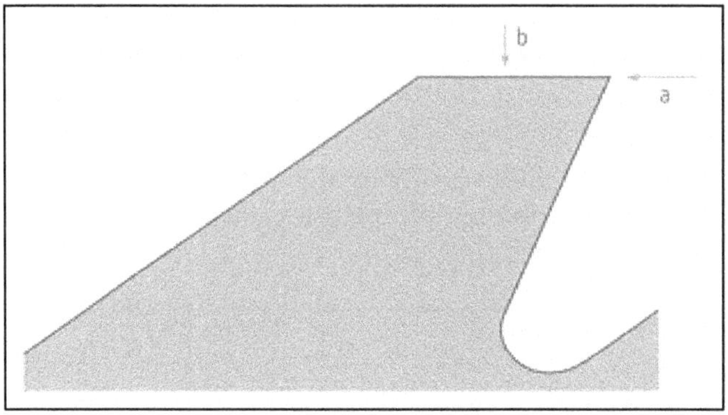

Figure 8.7: 'Hand' Area in Wire.

must only be ground down to a given depth, otherwise land (b) becomes too large and satisfactory carding is impossible – the clothing has to be replaced.

7. The Base of the Tooth

The base is broader than the point in order to give the tooth adequate strength, and also to hold the individual windings apart. Various forms can be distinguished. In order to mount the wire, the normal profile ((a) for the licker-in, (b) for the cylinder) is either pressed into a groove milled into the surface of the licker-in (a) or is simply wound under high tension onto the plain cylindrical surface of the main cylinder (b). (d) represents a locked wire and (c) a chained wire. Both can be applied to a smooth surface on the licker-in; in this case a milled groove is no longer necessary.

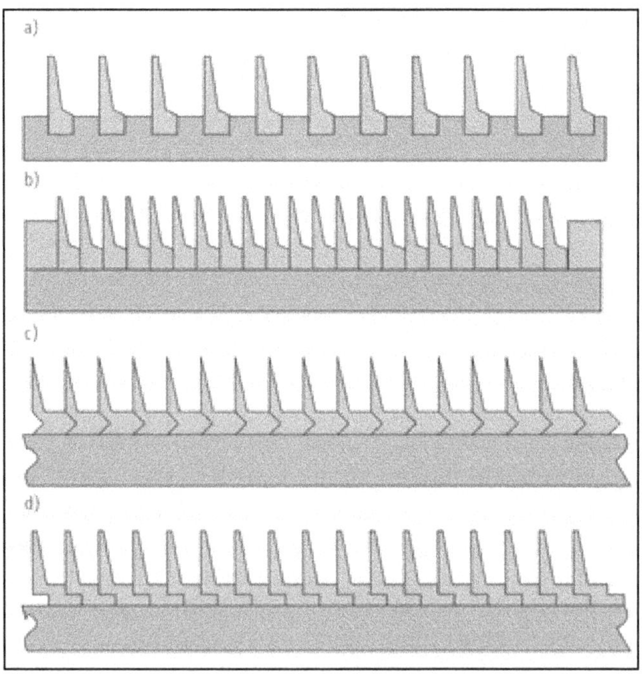

Figure 8.8: Formation of the Tooth Base and Mounting on the Drum.

8. Tooth hardness

In order to be able to process as much material as possible with one clothing, the tooth point must not wear away rapidly. Accordingly, a very hard point is needed, although it cannot be too hard because otherwise it tends to break off. On the other hand, to enable winding of the wire on a round body, the base must remain flexible. Each tooth therefore has to be hard at the tip and soft at the base.

Clothing Suggestions

C60 Card Clothing (Points / sq. inch - Front angle)					
Fibres	Very fine Yarn combed Ring	Med-Fine Yarn combed Nm 100	Coarse Yarn Carded / OE	Man Made > 1.0 dtex – 3.3	Man Made < 1.0 dtex – 0.6
Yarn count	> Nm 80 (>Ne 48)	Nm 40 .... 100 (Ne 24 .... 60)	< Nm 35 (< Ne 20)		
Production	50 kg/h		> 70 kg/h		
Licker-in - points	41	41 - 61	41 - 61	32	41
- angle	10 deg.	10 deg.	10 to 15 deg.	0 to 5 deg.	0 to 5 deg.
- rpm	1000 - 1350	1200 - 1600	1400 - 1800	?	1430
Example	Graf VE-5010V- -8	Graf VE-5010V- -8	Graf VE-5010V- -8	Graf VD-5005V- -8	Graf VE-5005V- -8
Cylinder - points	800 - 1080	965 to 1080	600 - 865	450 to 650	720
- angle	30 deg.	35 deg.	30 deg.	20 deg.	25 deg.
- rpm	750 - 850	800 - 850	850 - 900	600 - 750	600 - 700
Example	Graf P-2030 x 0.4 CS	Graf R1535 x 0.4	Graf R-2030 x 0.5	Graf R-2520 x 0.7	Graf P-2025 x 0.5
Flat clothing	550	550	410	350	430
Example	Graf RSTO F55/0	Graf RSTO F55/0	Graf RSTO C41/0	Graf ILXT M35/0	Graf PT 43/0
Doffer - points	340 - 365	340 - 365	280 - 340	280 - 340	340 - 365
- angle	30 deg.	30 deg.	30 deg.	30 deg.	30 deg.
Example	Graf N-4030B x 0.9	Graf M-5030 x 0.9	Graf L-4030B x 1.0	Graf L-4030B x 1.0	Graf M-5030 x 0.9

GRAF WIRE RECOMMENDATIONS

Clothing types for the widest range of requirements for various raw materials and card capacities are available. Below is a selection from our product range.

Production		Cotton			Man-made fibres (MMF)			Blends Co / MMF	Regenerates
		OE-yarn	carded	combed	< 1,0 dtex	1,5–3,0 dtex	> 3 dtex	or MMF 1,0–1,4 dtex	
< 15 kg/h	Cylinder	R-2525 x 0,6	R-2525 x 0,6	R-2530 x 0,6	R-2520 x 0,6	R-2515 x 0,7	O-3215 x 0,9	R-2520 x 0,6	R-2525 x 0,6
				R-2530 x 0,5					
	Doffer	N-4025B x 0,9	N-4025B x 0,9	N-4025B x 0,9	N-4025B x 0,9R	N-4025B x 0,9R	N-4025B x 0,9R	N-4025B x 0,9R	N-4025B x 0,9R
15–40 kg/h	Cylinder	R-2030 x 0,5	R-2030 x 0,5	R-2530 x 0,5	R-2525 x 0,6	R-2520 x 0,7	O-2515 x 0,9	R-2525 x 0,6	R-2525 x 0,6
		R-2030 x 0,6	R-2030 x 0,6	R-2030 x 0,5					R-2530 x 0,6
		R-2530 x 0,6	R-2530 x 0,6	P-2030 x 0,4					
	Doffer	N-4025B x 0,9	N-4025B x 0,9	N-4025B x 0,9	N-4025B x 0,9R	N-4025B x 0,9R	N-4025B x 0,9R	N-4025B x 0,9R	N-4030B x 0,9R
> 40 kg/h	Cylinder	R-2030 x 0,5	R-2030 x 0,5	R-2030 x 0,5	P-2025 x 0,5	R-2520 x 0,7	O-2515 x 0,9	R-2525 x 0,6	R-2525 x 0,6
		P-1840S x 0,4	P-2040S x 0,4	P-2030 x 0,4				P-2025 x 0,5	R-2530 x 0,5
		P-2040S x 0,4							R-2530 x 0,6
	Doffer	N-4030B x 0,9	N-4030B x 0,9	N-4030B x 0,9	N-4030B x 0,9R	N-4030B x 0,9R	N-4030B x 0,9R	N-4030B x 0,9R	N-4030B x 0,9R
		L-4030B x 1,0	L-4030B x 1,0						
	Lickerin	E-5510 x 1...	E-5510 x 1...	E-5510 x 1...	E-5505 x 1...	D-5505 x 1...	C-5500 x 1...	D-5505 x 1...	E-5510 x 1...
		V.E-5010V--8	V.E-5010V--8	V.E-5010V--8	V.E-5005V--8	V.D-5005V--8	V.C-5000V--8	V.D-5005V--8	V.E-5010V--8
		V.E-5010V-12	V.E-5010V-12		V.E-5005V-12				V.E-5010V-12

Production		Cotton			Man-made fibres (MMF)			Blends Co / MMF		Regenerates
		OE-yarn	carded	combed	< 1,0 dtex	1,5–3,0 dtex	> 3 dtex	Blends Co / MMF	MMF 1,0–1,4 dtex	
< 15 kg/h	PRIMATOP	PT 40/0-5		SPACETOP						
		PT 43/0	PT 43/0	PT 43/0	PT 43/0			PT 43/0		PT 40/0-5
	InLine-X-Top ILXT	C-40/0	C 40/0	F-50/0	M-40/0	M-35/0	M-35/0	C-40/0	M-40/0	C-40/0-7
	SUPRATOP					ST 35/0			ST 35/0	
	DIAMANT/PICCO-DIAMANT					DI/PD 33/0	DI/PD 24/0		DI/PD 33/0	
15–40 kg/h	PRIMATOP	PT 40/0-5								
		PT 43/0	PT 43/0	SPACETOP	PT 43/0			PT 43/0		PT 40/0-5
	InLine-X-Top ILXT	C-40/0	C-40/0	F-50/0	M-40/0	M-35/0	M-35/0	C-40/0	M-40/0	C-40/0-7
	SUPRATOP					ST 35/0			ST 35/0	
	resist-O-top RSTO	C-41/0	M-48/0	F-55/0				M-48/0		
	DIAMANT/PICCO-DIAMANT					DI/PD 33/0	DI/PD 24/0		DI/PD 33/0	
	M-TOP					MTM 31/0	MTM 31/0			
> 40 kg/h	PRIMATOP	PT 40/0-5								
		PT 43/0	PT 43/0	SPACETOP	PT 43/0			PT 43/0		PT 40/0-5
	InLine-X-Top ILXT	C-40/0	C-40/0	F-50/0	M-40/0	M-35/0	M-35/0	C-40/0	M-40/0	C-40/0-7
	SUPRATOP					ST 35/0			ST 35/0	
	resist-O-top RSTO	C-41/0	M-48/0	F-55/0				M-48/0		
	DIAMANT/PICCO-DIAMANT					DI/PD 33/0	DI/PD 24/0		DI/PD 33/0	
	M-TOP					MTM 31/0	MTM 31/0			MTR 42/0

WIRE POINT NOMENCLATURES

LCC WIRE

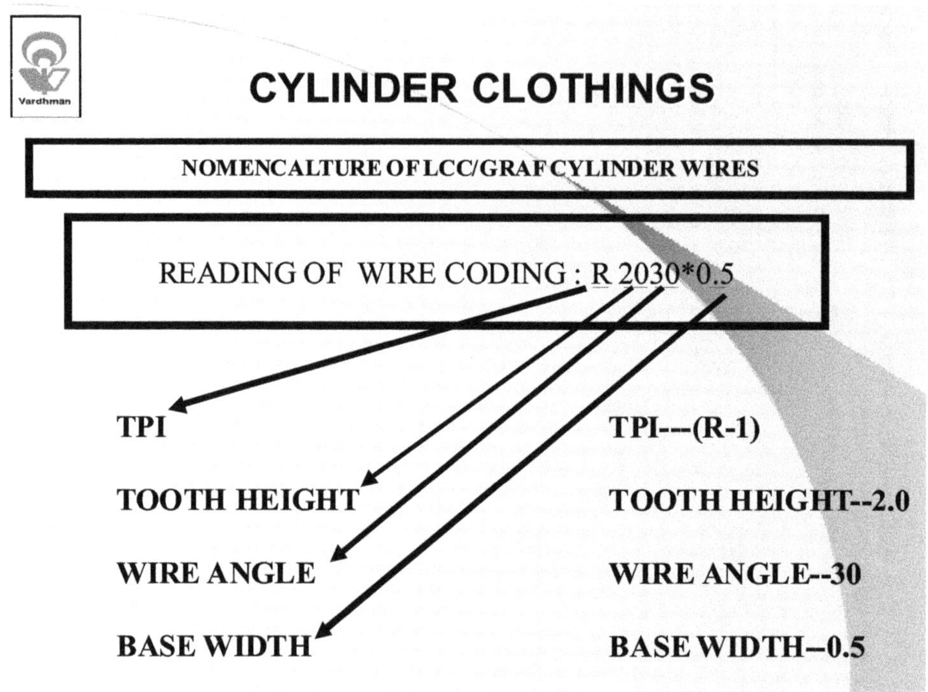

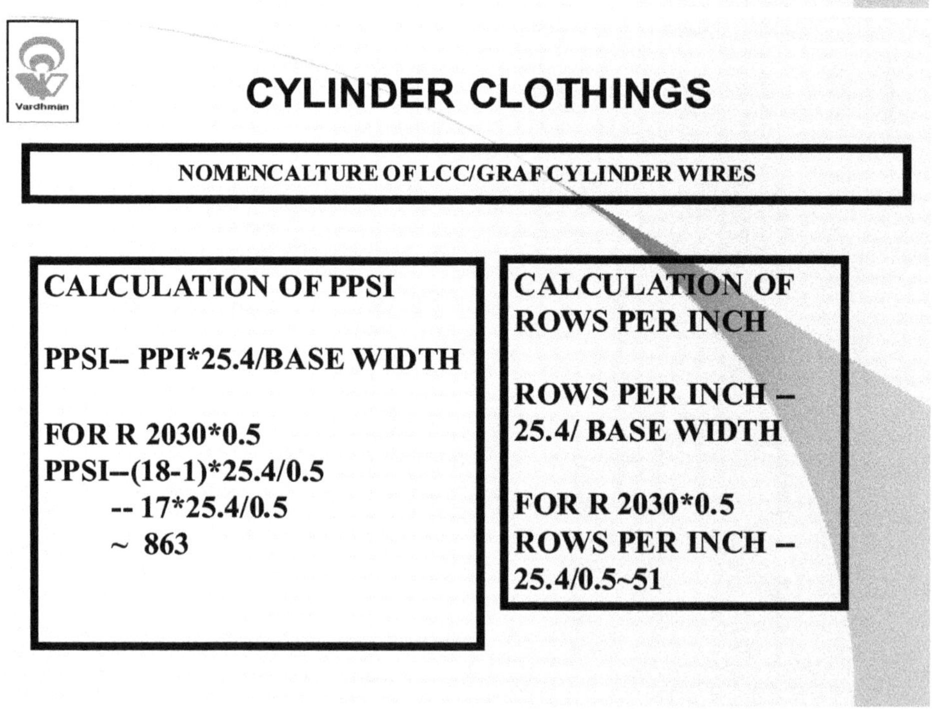

ICC WIRE

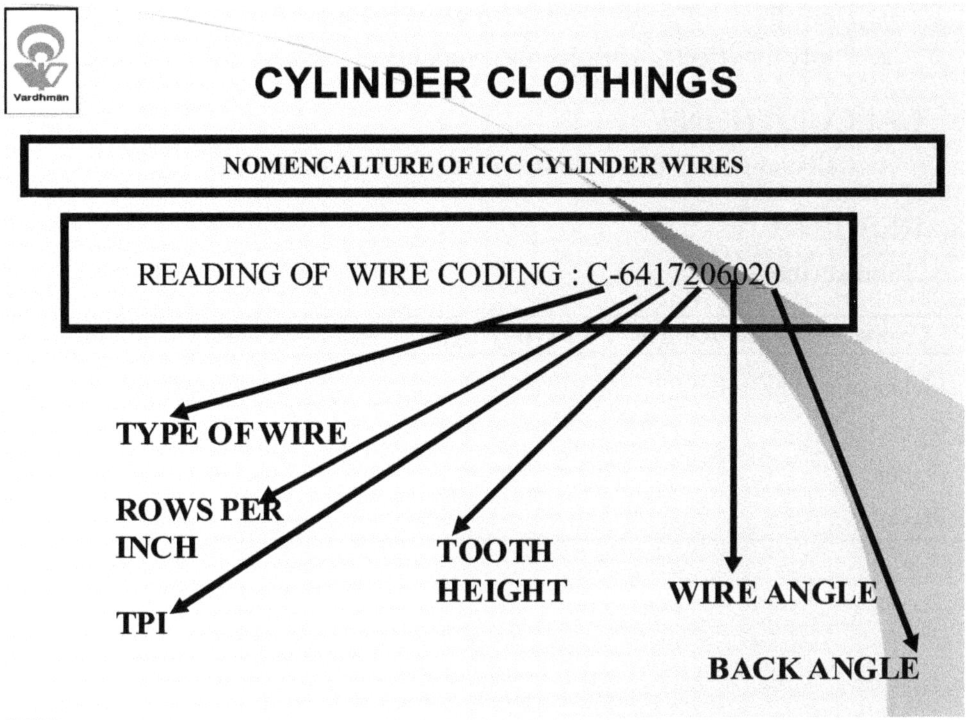

CYLINDER CLOTHINGS

NOMENCALTURE OF ICC CYLINDER WIRES

CALCULATION OF PPSI

PPSI-- ROWS PER INCH*PPI

FOR C-6417206020
PPSI--1088

CALCULATION OF BASE WIDTH

BASE WIDTH--25.4/ROWS PER INCH

FOR C-6417206020
BASE WIDTH--25.4/64~0.40

4. PROCEDURE

1. Draw the wire profile of the card wire clothing
2. Study the effect of wire profile on quality of yarn.

5. CALCULATIONS

1. Calculate the PPSI of cylinder, doffer and licker-in wires

6. RESULTS

Tabulate the results.

Component	*Wire Angle*	*Wire Height*	*Front Wire Angle*	*PPSI*
Licker-in				
Cylinder				
Doffer				
Flats				

9

Determination of Transfer–Coefficient and Cleaning Efficiency of Carding Machine

1. AIM

- ☆ To study the types of wire dispositions in carding machine.
- ☆ To study the fibre transfer mechanism between cylinder and doffer.
- ☆ To run the machine and calculate the cleaning efficiency of the carding machine.

2. FORMULA

Refer spinning useful formula relevant to your experiment

3. DESCRIPTION

Carding Action

This action is a fibre separation process from fibre tufts held in between two interacting wire covered surfaces (Figure 9.1).

The necessary conditions or carding are:

1. There should be two wire-covered surfaces facing each other. The distance between them at their closest approach should be around 0.3 mm or less (Nearly 20 to 30 times the fibre diameter).
2. The wires of both the interacting surfaces should be inclined in such a way that the point or tip of wire from one surface should face the point or tip of

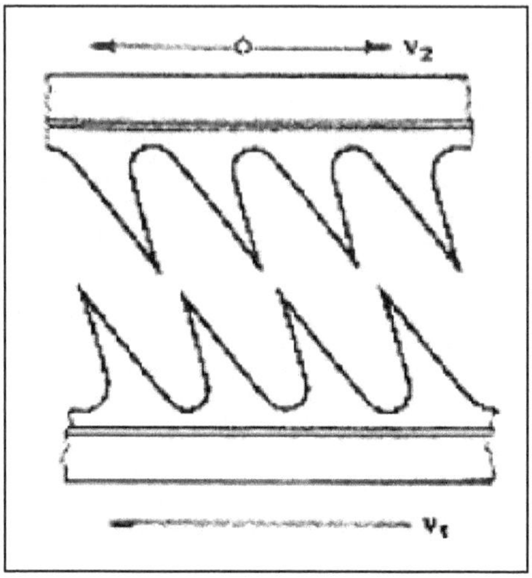

Figure 9.1: Point to Point Action.

the wire from the other clothed surface (point to point arrangement or carding disposition).

3. The interacting surfaces should move either in same or opposite direction at the point of interaction. If they move in the same direction, the surface charged with fibre (the surface, which brings the fibre) should move at higher linear velocity than the other surface in the direction in which their wire points are inclined.

Stripping Action

This action is a fibre transfer process from one wire surface to the other.

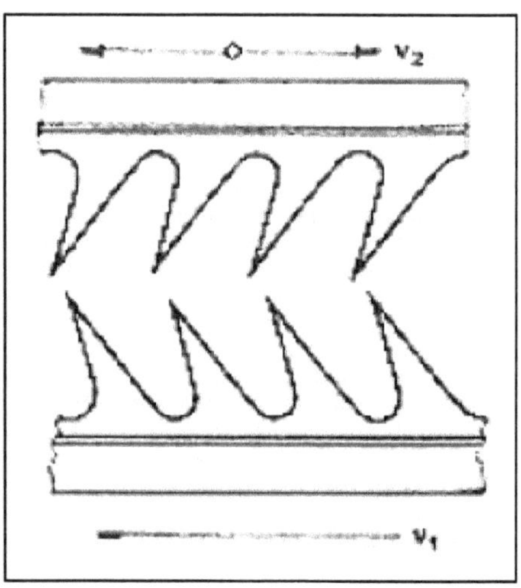

Figure 9.2: Point to Back Action.

The necessary conditions for stripping action of fibres are:

1. There should be two wire-covered surfaces facing each other. The distance between them at their closest approach should be around 0.3 mm or less. (Nearly 20 to 30 times the fibre diameter)
2. The wires of both the interfacing surfaces should be inclined in such a way that the point or tip of wire from one surface should face the back of the wire from the other clothed surface. (Point to back arrangement or doffing disposition)
3. The interacting surfaces should move either in same or opposite direction at the point of interaction. If they move in the same direction, the linear velocity of the surface on which the fibre is to be transferred, should be higher than the other surface charged with fibre.

FIBRE TRANSFER FROM CYLINDER TO DIFFER

The fibres are removed from the cylinder by the "doffer". They rotate so that the cylinder and doffer surfaces move in the same direction at the transfer zone.

- ☆ The doffer rotates at a considerably slower surface speed than does the cylinder and consequently fibres accumulate on the doffer wire.
- ☆ The doffer speed is normally in range of 50 to 120 m / min and the cylinder surface speed is in the region of 1500 m / min.
- ☆ The doffer takes some of the fibres carried by the cylinder, but the majority stays on the cylinder. There is a transfer factor in the order of 0.2 to 0.3,
- ☆ Fibres, on average, pass around the cylinder 3 to 5 times.
- ☆ The fibres taken up by the doffer are caught (hooked) on the wire and partially combed out by the passing cylinder wire. Consequently the fibres on the doffer have a majority of "trailing" hooks relative to the movement of the doffer and subsequent sliver.
- ☆ The fibres taken up by the doffer have to be held securely by the wire and must not drop from the wire as the doffer rotates.

The fibre transfer factor largely depends upon:

- ☆ The setting of the doffer to the cylinder,
- ☆ The type of doffer and cylinder clothing,
- ☆ The wire tooth geometry, particularly of the doffer,
- ☆ The number of points on the cylinder and doffer,
- ☆ The sharpness of the doffer wire,
- ☆ The aerodynamics at the exit region of the cylinder doffer zone.

ASSISTING FACTORS IN THE TRANSFER OF FIBRES FROM CYLINDER TO DOFFER

- ☆ The doffer continuously presents a clean surface to the cylinder at the point of interaction.

- ☆ The clothing on the doffer is usually 10 counts finer than that on the cylinder and the increases number of points per square inch increases the retentive power of the doffer clothing
- ☆ Owing to the curvature of the cylinder and doffer, the working surfaces move rapidly apart after the transfer of fibres to the doffer, so that there is little opportunity for the return of fibres to the cylinder.
- ☆ Centrifugal force due to the high cylinder speed tends to throw fibres towards the doffer, whereas the much lower speed of the latter prevents corresponding forces in the reverse direction.
- ☆ Air currents may also assist the transfer of fibres to the doffer.

Hook Formation

The doffer clothing has a limited filling capacity. It depends upon the fibre fineness and for a one-meter wide card is limited to about 3 to 5 g/m (42 to70 grains/ yard). When the filling approaches or exceeds maximum loading, the extra fibre tends to be entangled and produces a cloudy web. This cloudy characteristic has poor fibre orientation and produces a weak web that can be difficult to control. With short staple fibres this cloudiness can be drafted out in the drawing processes and will have only a limited effect.

However, with long staple fine fibres the extra web material responds to the drawing process by forming an excessive number of knots or neps. This phenomenon occurs with both long staple cotton and fine man-made fibres. In general, lighter web weights/cm² are better than heavier web weights for quality spinning.

As mentioned earlier, in the doffing process, the fibres are hooked around the doffer wire and this creates "trailing" hooks. According to Morton and Yen the percentages of the various fibre shapes in the card sliver are as follows:

Typical fibre shapes in the card sliver		
Designation	Shape	Approx. %
Trailing hooks	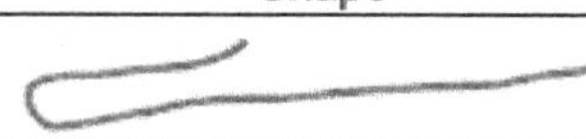	Over 50%
Leading hooks	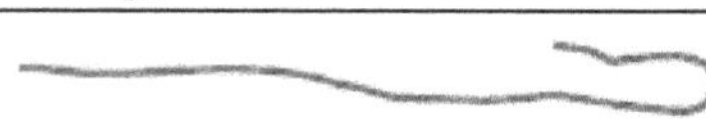	15%
Double hooks	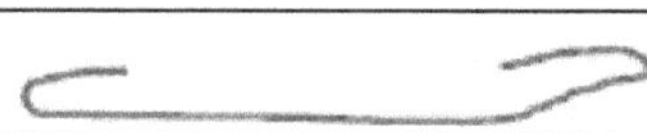	15%
No hooks	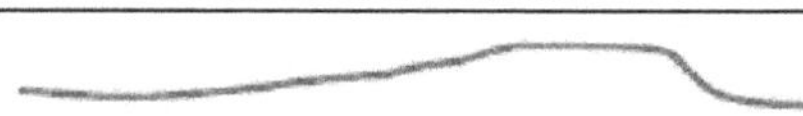	20%
Direction of movement →		

Figure 9.3: Types of Fibre Hooks in Card Sliver.

THEORY OF TRANSFER-COEFFICIENT

The fibre layer carried to the doffer will be split up in to two parts. If the doffer splits away and retains say ½ of the layer this will pass out from the card. The remaining half remains on the cylinder and after about half a revolution will be joined by a new unit "feed quantity" of fibre transferred to it by the feed roll/licker-in assembly. These fibres are more or less individualized by the time they reach the doffer.

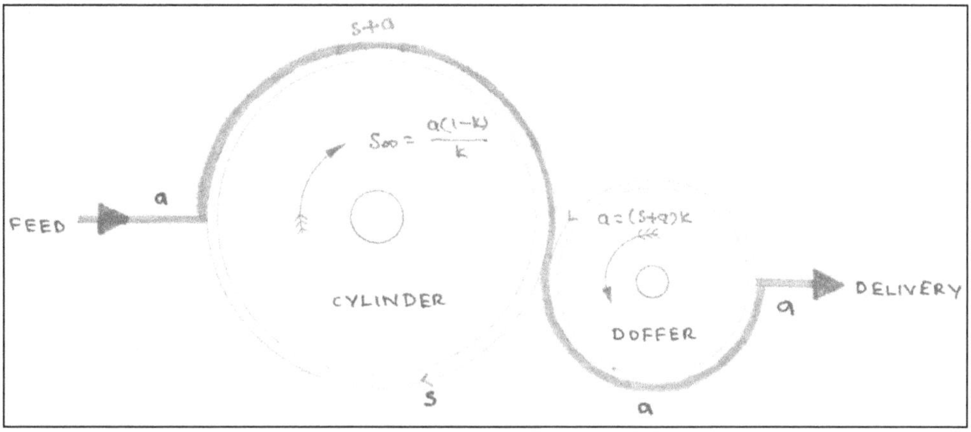

Figure 9.4: Transfer-Coefficient

The splitting and retaining power of the doffer is called "Transfer Coefficient". Thus, if total volume of fibres were to be retained by a doffer its TC would be 1; if only half of the fibres were retained, the TC would be 0.5; if only one quarter of the fibres retained, the TC would be 0.25 and so on.

Let it be assumed that,

☆ The quantity of fibres fed into the card	= a
☆ If, TC of the doffer	= k
☆ In one revolution the doffer retained of fibres	= a x k
☆ Leaving a quantity on the cylinder	= a(1-k)
☆ During the next revolution, the cylinder receives again a fresh quantity	= a
☆ Now the total fibres on the cylinder surface	= a + a(1-k)
☆ The doffer splits away	= (a + a(1-k))k
☆ Leaving the fibres on the cylinder	= (a + a(1-k)) x (1-k)

Thus the quantity of retained fibres on the cylinder goes on increasing until a limit is reached, the cylinder is saturated and the fibre distribution on the card is in equilibrium.

The total load "S" on the cylinder after "n" revolution of the offer is

$Sn = a\,(1 + (1-k) + (1-k^2) + (1-k^3) + \ldots\ldots\ldots\ldots + (1-k^n)$

The total sum to infinity can be written as:

$$S_{\propto} = \frac{a(1-k)}{k}, \text{ Equilibrium of the card.}$$

Let us take an example:

If feed per doffer revolution (a) = 1

The retaining capacity of the doffer (k) = 10% is 0.1

Then the saturated fibre load of cylinder $S_{\propto} = \frac{a(1-k)}{k}$

$= 1(1\text{-}0.1)/0.1 = 9$

After one more revolution of the doffer $S_{\propto} + a = 9 + 1 = 10$

4. PROCEDURE

1. Clean the machine thoroughly in order to keep flats, cylinder and doffer surfaces free from fibres.
2. Take a lap, place it on the lap roller and then engage the lap end with the feed roller
3. Start the machine. Once the card attains steady state (normally it takes 3-4 minutes), stop only doffer, which usually results in stopping the feed also.
4. Cut off drive to feed roller and flats
5. Restart the doffer again. At first the fibres already lying on the doffer surface in the region between doffer comb and the junction between the cylinder and doffer will come out, followed by fibres left on the operational layer of cylinder. One can notice a clear dividing line between the two.
6. Weigh the fibres from the dividing line to the cessation of fibre delivery which is an approximate estimation of Q.
7. Measure the linear density of the sliver produced during steady state.
8. Note down cylinder and doffer speed.

5. CALCULATIONS

Transfer co-efficient is defined as the% of fibre in weight transferred from the operational layer of cylinder to doffer per revolution of the cylinder. Mathematically,

$$k = \frac{q}{Q} \times 100$$

where,

q = Amount of fibre (gm) transferred to doffer per revolution of cylinder

Q = Load on the operational layer of cylinder at steady state

During the revolution of cylinder the length of sliver (L) delivered by doffer is

$$L = \frac{1}{n_c} \times \Pi \times D_d \times n_d$$

where,

D_d = Doffer dia

n_d = Doffer speed

n_c = Cylinder speed

If h is the count of sliver (n_c), then the weight of sliver (q) delivered on one revolution of cylinder,

$$q = \frac{453.67 \times \Pi \times D_d \times n_d}{h \times 840 \times n_c \times 36}$$

$$k = \frac{453.67 \times \Pi \times D_d \times n_d}{h \times 840 \times n_c \times 36} \times \frac{100}{Q}$$

In order to determine k, Q has been found experimentally.

Cleaning Efficiency

1. Take the sample of cotton from blow room lap or from the feed of the card.
2. Find out the trash% in lap using Shirley Trash Analyzer
3. Run the machine and Take the sample of cotton card sliver from the output.
4. Find out the trash% in card sliver using Shirley Trash Analyzer
5. Calculate the Cleaning Efficiency of the card using the formula:

$$\text{Cleaning Efficiency} = \frac{\text{Trash \% in lap} - \text{Trash \% in sliver}}{\text{Trash \% in lap}} \times 100$$

6. RESULTS

Tabulate the results.

10

Construction and Working Mechanism of Draw Frame Machine

1. AIM

- ✰ To draw the gearing diagram of the machine
- ✰ To observe the design features and important functional elements of the machine / mechanism
- ✰ To calculate the delivery rate in mpm, Individual draft, Total draft and Production of the machine in Kgs / Shift.
- ✰ To identify the Draft Change Wheel (DCW)

2. FORMULA

Refer spinning useful formula relevant to your experiment

3. DESCRIPTION

The Task of Draw Frame

Equalizing

One of the main tasks of the drawframe is improving evenness over the short, medium and – especially – long term. Card slivers fed to the drawframe have a degree of unevenness that cannot be tolerated in practice, and slivers from the comber contain the „infamous" piecings; these must be obscured. It should be noted, however, that short-wave sliver evenness is not – as sometimes assumed – the sole criterion for evaluating the performance of the drawframe. It is true, for example, that unevenness over short lengths can be noticeably reduced, *e.g.* by very narrow setting of the rollers of the drafting arrangement, but this is often associated with deterioration in other quality parameters of the yarn, particularly strength.

It is also a mistake to assume that sliver evenness – especially over short lengths – can be significantly improved by using several passages. A second passage brings hardly any improvement and a third can actually lead to deterioration. In relation to settings and number of passages, therefore, it is important to find the optimum rather than seek the maximum. Equalizing is always and in any case performed by doubling, and can optionally also be performed by additional autolevelling. The draft and the doublings often have the same value and are in the range of 6 (short fibers) to 8 (medium and long fibers). When processing pure comber noil in the rotor spinning mill, however, it is usually necessary to settle for a value of 4 or to use high-performance cards with integrated levelling devices instead of draw frames.

Parallelizing

To obtain an optimal value for strength in the yarn characteristics, the fibers must be arranged parallel in the fiber strand. It is mainly the draw frame's task to create this parallel arrangement. It fulfills this task by means of the draft, since every drafting step leads to straightening of the fibers. The value of the draft must be adapted to the material, *i.e.* to several fiber parameters, mainly:

- ☆ The staple length;
- ☆ The mass of the fibers;
- ☆ The volume of the strand;
- ☆ The degree of order (parallel disposition).

It will be clear that the draft cannot be high on a machine directly following the card (if possible, not above 8), but thereafter can increase from machine to machine.

Blending

In addition to the equalizing effect, doubling also provides a degree of compensation of raw material variations by blending, which occurs simultaneously. This result is exploited in particular in the production of blended yarns comprising cotton / synthetic or synthetic / synthetic blends. At the drawframe, metering of the individual components can be carried out very simply by selection of the number of slivers entering the machine. For example, to obtain a 67:33 blend, four slivers of one component and two of the other are fed to the drawframe. Of course, these slivers must have the same hank.

Dust Removal

Dust is steadily becoming a greater problem both in processing and for the personnel involved. It is therefore important to remove dust to the greatest practical extent at every possible point within the overall process. Unfortunately, dust removal can only be carried out to a significant degree when there are high levels of fiber / fiber or fiber / metal friction, since a large proportion of these very small particles (dust) adhere relatively strongly to the fibers. Such friction arises especially on the card and the drawframe; in the latter case, mainly owing to the drafting operation. The drawframe is therefore a good dust-removing machine. On high-performance draw frames equipped with appropriate suction systems, more than 80% of the incoming dust is extracted.

Operating Principle

Four to eight card or drawframe slivers are fed to the drafting arrangement (**3**). A feed roller pair (**2**) is located above each can (**1**) to enable the feeding step to be performed in a controlled manner without false drafts. In some cases (seldom) a simple deflection bar is sufficient. The feed roller pairs are mounted in a creel frame or table and each is positively driven. The slivers running into the drafting arrangement leave it, after a draft of 4 to 8, as a web lacking significant cohesion. In order to avoid disintegration of the web, which would otherwise be unavoidable at the high operating speeds currently in use, it is condensed into a sliver immediately after the drafting arrangement. This sliver is then (for example in some makes) guided through a tube (**4**) via a passage (**6**) of the tube gear into a can (**7**), in which it must be laid in clean coils with optimal utilization of the space in the can. To enable the can to take up as much material as possible, the sliver is compressed by passing it through calendering rollers (or discs) or grooved discs (**5**).

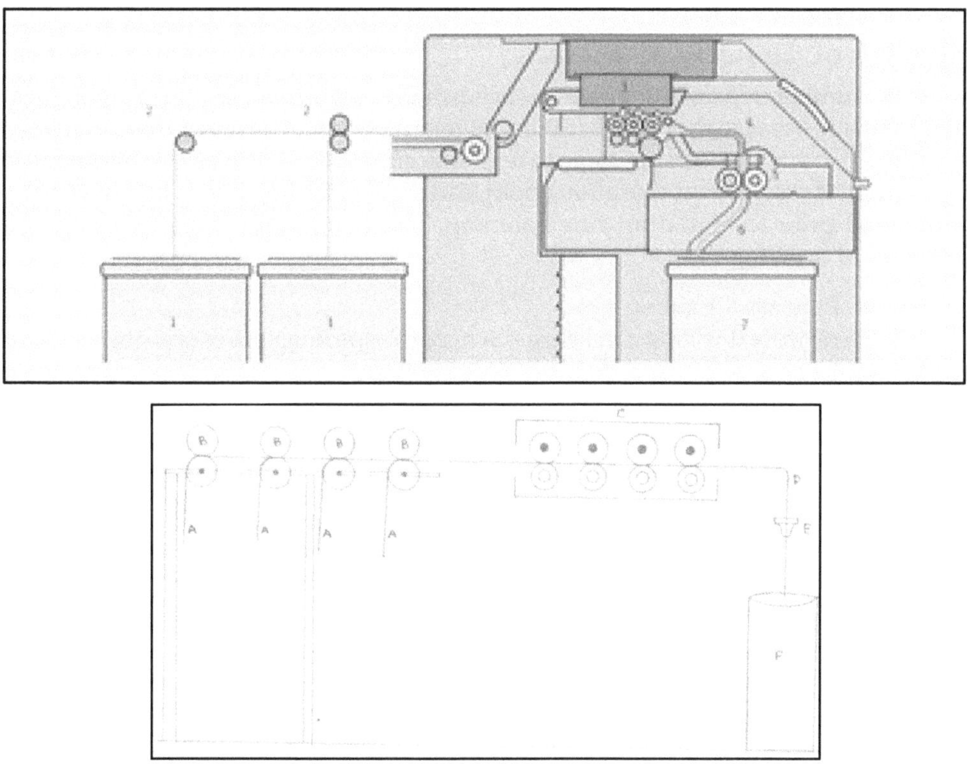

Figure 10.1: Sectional View of a Drawframe.

A: Card slivee; B: Careel guide roller; C: 4/4 drafting system; D: Drafted sliver; E: Trumpet; F: Delivery can.

Influence of Fibres

The basic rules are:

- ☆ Long, fine fibres of uniform length can be drafted at the high end of the draft range, carded cotton and blends should be limited to a maximum draft of eight.
- ☆ With very short regenerated fibres the draft should be limited to four, and only one process of drawing. Multiple drawing processes create a very high level of drafting waves. Additionally, these fibres normally have to be run at speeds below 400 m/min.
- ☆ Synthetic fibres with high fibre-to-fibre cohesion require higher drafting forces, create more heat and in general have to run at slower speed, in the range of 400 to 500 m/min.
- ☆ The fibre finish on some synthetic fibres can create a finish build up on the machine, in the coiler tube and on the coiler plate. Care has to be taken to keep the machine clean.
- ☆ Some bulky synthetic fibres need special components to run well. Check with the business unit if this is a problem.

Number of Drawing Processes

The number of drawing processes is normally established by the technological requirements because the cost of drawing is relatively low. However, there is always pressure to reduce processing steps to remain competitive. It is well established that the card produces a sliver containing both leading and trailing hooks that have to be eliminated prior to high draft ring spinning. This is normally done by using two passages of drawing.

1. Single Process Drawing

Single process drawing can be used where the spinning process is not sensitive to fibre hooks or poor fibre orientation. These include:

- ☆ The spinning of coarse counts from blends containing very short fibres such as comber noil, regenerated fibres or gin motes. An additional drawing process is not used with this type of material because it can create problems of drafting waves and reduced sliver cohesion.
- ☆ Rotor spinning of coarse and some medium count yarns. Fibre hooks and fibre orientation do not greatly affect the spinning process but there will be a loss of strength by using only one process of drawing. This is not a problem for many applications.
- ☆ Coarse counts spun from synthetic fibres. Some carpet and upholstery yarns are produced on both ring and rotor spinning systems.

2. Two Process Drawing

The conventional short staple process, for "carded" yarns of cotton, man made fibres and intimate blends, includes two drawing processes. The primary reasons for two processes are:

- To reduce the number of fibre hooks in the sliver,
- Supply roving, with the majority of hooks trailing, to the ring spinning,
- To improve the degree of fibre orientation in the sliver,
- To enable blending through doubling to improve yarn consistency,
- To gradually reduce the sliver weight from the card sliver to that needed by the roving or spinning machines.

Drawing for Combed Yarns

In the modern combed yarn spinning, there are three drawing operations:

- First passage of preparation drawing is used to draw card sliver and produce sliver that can be wound onto laps for the comber.
- The second drawing operation occurs at the comber to reduce the sliver weight. Relatively high drafts are needed at this stage and the drafting zone is very robust. The drafting system is normally a 3 over 5 roller arrangement to clearly separate the fibre control function of the break draft zone and the main draft zone.
- The third drawing operation is performed on the finisher Drawframe.
- The comber eliminates most of the fibre hooks, hence the remaining functions of the Drawframe are to produce a very uniform sliver of the required weight. This "one process drawing" after combing has been made possible by the successful use of the RSB autoleveller Drawframe.

6. CALCULATIONS

1. Calculate the speed of drafting rollers.
2. Calculate the individual draft, total draft and draft constant
3. Calculate the production of the machine.

7. RESULTS

Tabulate the results.

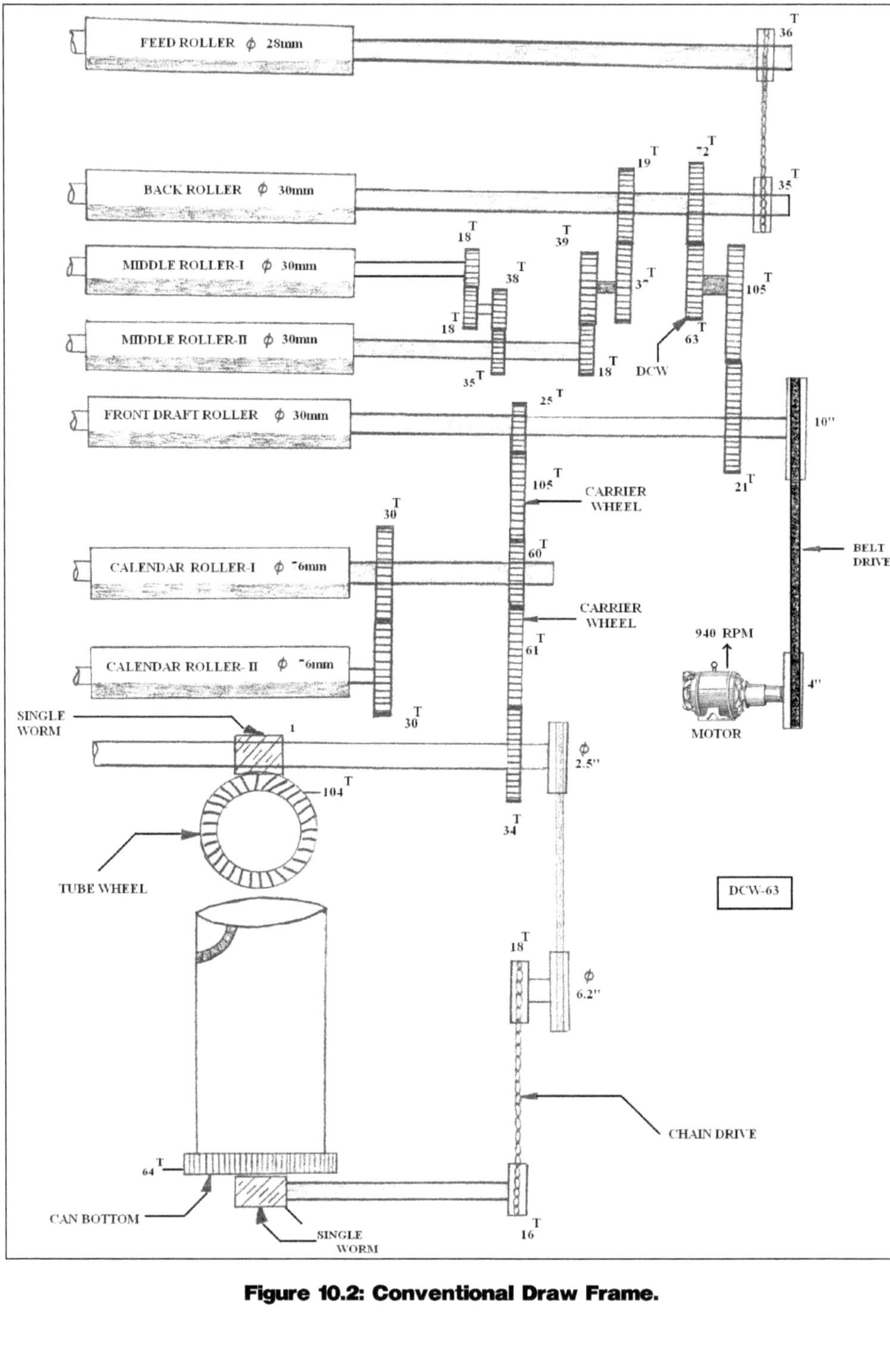

Figure 10.2: Conventional Draw Frame.

11

Determination of Total Draft and its Distribution in Draw Frame Drafting System

1. AIM

- ☆ To draw the gearing diagram of the machine
- ☆ To observe the design features and important functional elements of the machine / mechanism
- ☆ To calculate the delivery rate in mpm, Individual draft, Total draft and Production of the machine in Kgs / Shift.
- ☆ To identify the Draft Change Wheel (DCW)

2. FORMULA

Refer spinning useful formula relevant to your experiment

3. DESCRIPTION

Drafting Arrangements

The drafting arrangement is the heart of the drawframe and thus the part which exerts the most decisive influence on quality. The requirements placed on the drafting arrangement in general are correspondingly high:

- ☆ Simple, uncomplicated construction;
- ☆ Stable design with smooth running of the rollers (centricity);

- ☆ A mode of operation producing a high-quality product even at high running speeds;
- ☆ High degree of flexibility, *i.e.* suitability for all raw materials, fiber lengths, sliver hanks, etc., that might be processed in the short staple spinning mill;
- ☆ Optimal control over the movement of the fibers during the drafting operation;
- ☆ High precision of both operation and adjustment;
- ☆ Rapid and simple adjustability of roller spacings and draft levels;
- ☆ Ease of maintenance and cleaning;
- ☆ Optimal ergonomic design.

Influences on the Draft

In all types of drafting arrangement, the factors that affect the draft are:

Factors dependent upon the fiber material:

- ☆ Mass of fiber in the strand cross section;
- ☆ Degree of order of the fibers (parallel disposition);
- ☆ Shape of the cross section of the fiber strand;
- ☆ Compactness of the fiber strand;
- ☆ Adhesion between the fibers dependent upon
- ☆ Surface structure,
- ☆ Crimp,
- ☆ Spin finish,
- ☆ Compression of the strand;
- ☆ Fiber length;
- ☆ Evenness of distribution of fiber lengths (staple form);
- ☆ Existing twist in the fiber strand.

Factors dependent upon the drafting arrangement:

- ☆ Diameter of the rollers;
- ☆ Hardness of the top rollers;
- ☆ Pressure exerted by the top rollers;
- ☆ Surface characteristics of the top rollers;
- ☆ Fluting of the bottom rollers;
- ☆ Type and form of fiber guiding devices, such as pressure rods, pin bars, aprons, condenser etc.;
- ☆ Clamping distances (roller settings);
- ☆ Level of draft;
- ☆ Distribution of draft between the various drafting zones.

Drafting System

The drafting system is basically 3 over 3 with an additional "Deflection" roll (7) on the delivery roll to direct the sliver toward the coiler. The top rolls are numbered (1, 2, 3) and corresponding bottom rolls are, - back roll (4), middle roll (5) and delivery roll (6). There is a pressure bar (8) located between the top rolls 2 and 3 to help control the fibres in the main draft zone. The fundamental settings of the drafting system are the roll distances and the draft distribution. Each greatly influences the quality of the delivered sliver.

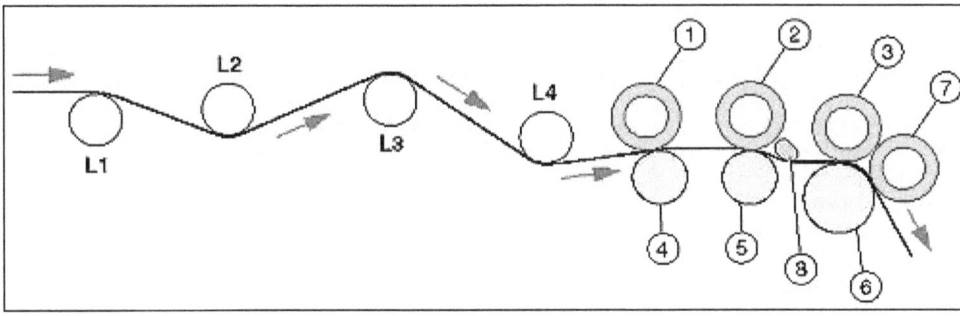

Figure 11.1: Draw Frame Drafting System.

Draft Distribution

- ☆ The total draft is established by the total mass of the input material and the mass of the output sliver.
- ☆ The calculation is: Total draft (V) = Input mass / Delivered mass

The total draft is performed in two stages. The first step is the "Break Draft" (V V), which prepares the slivers for the "Main Draft" (V H)

Break Draft Zone – Draft (V V)

The function of the break draft in the Drawframe is to pre tension the slivers and remove the sliver crimp so that the fibres presented to the main draft zone are controlled. The normal range is 1.16 to 1.41, but with polyester for sewing thread and crimped acrylic the break draft can be up to 1.70. The break draft in the first drawing passage is usually higher than that of the second passage because the card sliver has a lower level of fibre orientation. The evenness tester diagram and spectrogram should be used as a guide in setting the draft. The following observations can be made:

- ☆ Breaker drawing requires higher break draft than subsequent drawing processes.
- ☆ Warning: Roll settings that are too close will result in over control, which can be seen as "spikes" in the evenness diagram. These spikes cause thick and thin places in the yarn.
- ☆ Finisher drawing requires more open settings and a lower break draft.
- ☆ Man made fibres require higher break drafts than cotton.

- ✰ Finer fibres, cotton or man made, require higher break draft than coarser fibres.
- ✰ When the total draft has to be relatively high (7 to 10) the break draft has to be increased to keep the main draft in the desirable range.
- ✰ When processing short fibres the break draft should be low.

Main Draft Zone – Draft (HV)

The main draft is established by the total draft and the break draft. The total draft is set by the overall processing system and usually has to be accepted. However, for high quality products, it is recommended to limit the Drawframe draft to less than eight (8), which means the main draft will be between 3.5 and 5.5.

Suction Systems for the Drafting Arrangement

One of the tasks of the drawframe is dust removal. Release of dust occurs almost exclusively in the drafting arrangement and this should be totally enclosed so that dust does not pass into the surrounding atmosphere. The dust-laden air must be extracted by suction (as shown in Figure). Each roller of the arrangement has an associated cleaning device (scraping bar and suction tube) so that fly and fibers tending to adhere to the rollers can also be carried away. In addition, on the Rieter drawframe the scraping bars are lifted from the top rollers intermittently. Trash collections therefore pass into the dust removal system. The air extracted is passed via tubes directly to filters within the machine and then into the exhaust ducts of the air-conditioning system or directly into those ducts. Filters within the machine are cleaned manually or by a wiper. This latter arrangement has the advantage not only of easier handling but also of constant suction pressure, resulting in constant cleaning efficiency.

The drafting action causes dust and flies to be released from the fibres. The airborne waste must be removed or it accumulates and eventually returns into the sliver as contamination. The integrated suction system removes dust and flies from the sliver:

- ✰ At the jockey rolls,
- ✰ The scanning rolls,
- ✰ Above the drafting system,
- ✰ Below the drafting system.

The integrated waste system is equipped with a pressure sensitive switch, which controls a wiper over the filter screen, to release waste accumulations. The Drawframe should be kept as clean as possible and periodic manual cleaning is necessary. The cleaning cycle depends upon the cleanliness of the material being processed. Bottom roll clearers have to be manually cleaned.

Tension Draft between Front Rolls and Calender Rolls

The tension draft between the front rolls and the calender rolls, (delivery rolls) will affect the running performance and the sliver quality. The tension has to be sufficient to gather the web and pull the sliver through the condenser in a controlled

Roll settings and draft recommendations

Material	Max. staple length mm	Process drawing	Doubling	Feed ktex	Total draft V	Break draft VV	Main draft roll setting HVD	Break draft roll setting VVD
100% comber noil	23	I RSB	4	6	4,9	1.28	35,5	37
Intimate blend 65% CO / 35% comber noil CO waste	38	I SB	4-6	4,5 - 6	4-6	1.16	37	37-38
		II RSB-D 30	4-6	4,5-6	4-6	1,16 (1,057)	37	37-38
CO carded, with high amount of short fibres	34	I SB	6	5	5-5,5	1,28	37,5	39
		II RSB-D 30	6	5	5-5,5	1,16	37,5	42
Peru Tanguis carded (_)= 8 doubling	spin-staple approx. 34...39	I SB	6-8	4,3	6-8	1,28 1,16	38	43 47
		II RSB-D 30	6 (8)	4,3	6 (8)	(1,28)	38	(44)
CO Combed 1 1/16"	36	I RSB-D 30	6	4,2	7,1	1,16	38	45
Egyptian CO, combed SL 2,5% = 34,6 mm SL 50% = 18,5 mm	38-39	I RSB-D 30	8	5,3	8	1,16	40	52
	43	I RSB-D 30	8	4,2	8,3	1,16	44	52
50% cotton combed 50% PES 1,7 dtex/ 40 mm	38/39	I/II SB	8	5	8	1,41 /1,28	43	48
		III RSB-D 30	8	5	8	1,28-1,41	44	50
50% cotton 1 1/16"carded 50% modal 1,3 dtex/ 38 mm	38	I/II SB	8	4	8	1,41	42	46
		III RSB-D 30	8	4	8	1,28	41	48
CV (viscose) 1,3/40 mm	38	I SB	8	4,9	9	1,41	43	46
		II RSB-D 30	8	4,7	8,3	1,28	44	48
PAC 1,3 dtex/ 40 mm crimped	38	I SB	6	4,6	6,8	1,70	44	48
		II RSB-D 30	6	4	6,7	1,28	44	50
PES 1,9 dtex/ 38 mm crimped	38	I SB	8	4,8	8,4	1,41	43	50
		II RSB-D 30	8	4,6	8	1,28	43	50
Sewing thread PES 1,3 dtex/ 38 mm	38	I SB	6	3,8	6,4	1,70	44	50
		II RSB-D 30	6	3,6	6,4	1,70	44	48
PAC 3,3 dtex/ 60 mm, crimped, dyed	spin staple approx. 53/54	I SB	6	5,0	6	1,70	58	65
		II RSB-D 30	6	5,0	8	1,41	58	65

Figure 11.2: Recommended Roller Settings and Draft in Draw Frame.

manner. However, if the tension is too high the sliver uniformity will deteriorate and the sliver Uster CV% can be 0.5% higher than it should be. As a guide, the following are tension ranges frequently used for different materials:

- ☆ Carded Cotton 1.01 to 1.02,
- ☆ Combed Cotton 1.00 to 1.01,
- ☆ Polyester/Cotton 0.99 to 1.0,
- ☆ 100% Synthetics 0.98 to 1.00

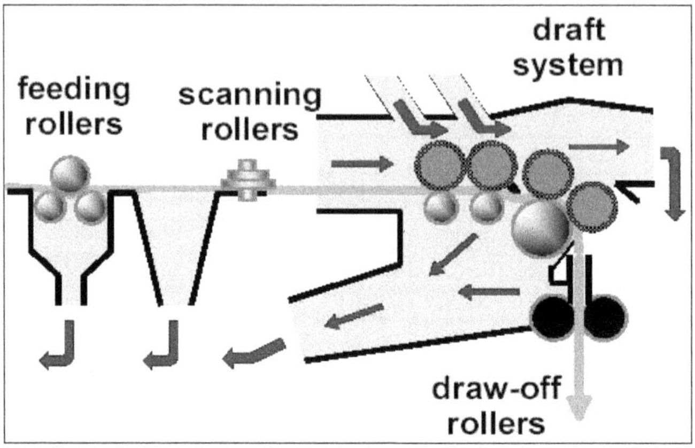

Figure 11.3: 4-over-3 Drafting Arrangement with Suction System.

Passage	Draft	Carded Cotton: With High percentage of Short fibres e.g. Noils	Carded Cotton: Normal Staple	Carded Cotton: With 50% Manmade fibres	Combed Cotton: 100%	Combed Cotton: With 50% Manmade fibres predrafted	Manmade fibres 100% 38/40mm	Manmade fibres 100% 50mm
1st	Total draft	3.4 – 5.6	5 – 8	6 – 8	6 – 8	6 – 8	6 – 9	6 – 8
	Prel. draft	1.16 (1.28)	1.28 (1.16) (1.41)*	1.16 – 1.28 (1.41)	1.16 (1.28)	1.16 – 1.28 (1.41)	1.41 (1.70)*	1.41 (1.70)*
2nd & 3rd	Total draft	3.4 – 5.5	5 – 8	6 – 8.5	-	6 – 8.5	6 – 9	5 – 8
	Prel. draft	1.16 (1.05)	1.16 (1.28)	1.16 – 1.28 (1.41)*	-	1.16 – 1.28 (1.41)	1.16 - 1.41 (1.70)*	1.28 - 1.41 (1.70)*

Figure 11.4

DRAFTING DESIGNATIONS

Draft

The draft in a drafting system may be defined as the ratio of length of sliver fed by the feed rollers to the length delivered by the delivery rollers per revolution of feed roller. Let the diameter of feed and delivery rollers be 'd' and 'D' respectively.

The amount fed per revolution of feed roller = Πd

The amount delivered per revolution of feed roller =

$$\frac{\Pi D \times \text{No. of revolution of delivery roller}}{\text{Revolution of feed roller}}$$

$$\text{Draft} = \frac{\Pi D \times \text{No. of revolution of delivery roller}}{\Pi D \times \text{Revolution of feed roller}}$$

Draft Constant

Draft constant is the magnitude of draft that one would obtain when the number of teeth of the draft change wheel (DCW) in a drafting system is considered to be one. Mathematically,

☆ Draft Constant = Draft x No. of teeth of DCW (when DCW become a driver gear when considering back roller as driver)

☆ Draft Constant = Draft / No. of teeth of DCW (when DCW becomes a driven)

Actual Draft

It is determined by taking the ratio of linear densities (in terms of Ne) of output sliver to that of combined input slivers.

$$\text{Actual Draft} = \frac{\text{Hank delivered}}{\text{Hank fed}}$$

4. PROCEDURE

1. Sketch the gearing diagram of the drafting system
2. Note down the number of teeth of various gears and measure the diameters of the bottom drafting rollers.
3. Mark the draft change wheel (DCW)
4. Select a can of sliver
5. Feed six sliver ends at the back and then run the machine for few minutes.

5. CALCULATION

1. Calculate the number of revolution of calendar roller per revolution of back roller
2. Calculate the number of revolution of 3rd roller per revolution of back roller
3. Calculate the number of revolution of 2nd roller per revolution of 3rd roller
4. Calculate the number of revolution of front roller per revolution of 2nd roller
5. Calculate the draft in the respective drafting zones using formula
6. Determine the count (in Ne) of feed and delivered slivers
7. Plot a graph showing draft as a function of number of teeth of DCW.

6. RESULTS

Zone	*Feed roller*	*Delivery roller*	*Draft*	*Draft Constant*
Creel Draft	Feed roller	Back		
Back zone	Back	4th		
Middle zone I	4th	3rd		
Middle zone II	3rd	2nd		
Front zone	2nd	1st		
Tension	1st	Calendar		
Total	Back	Calendar		

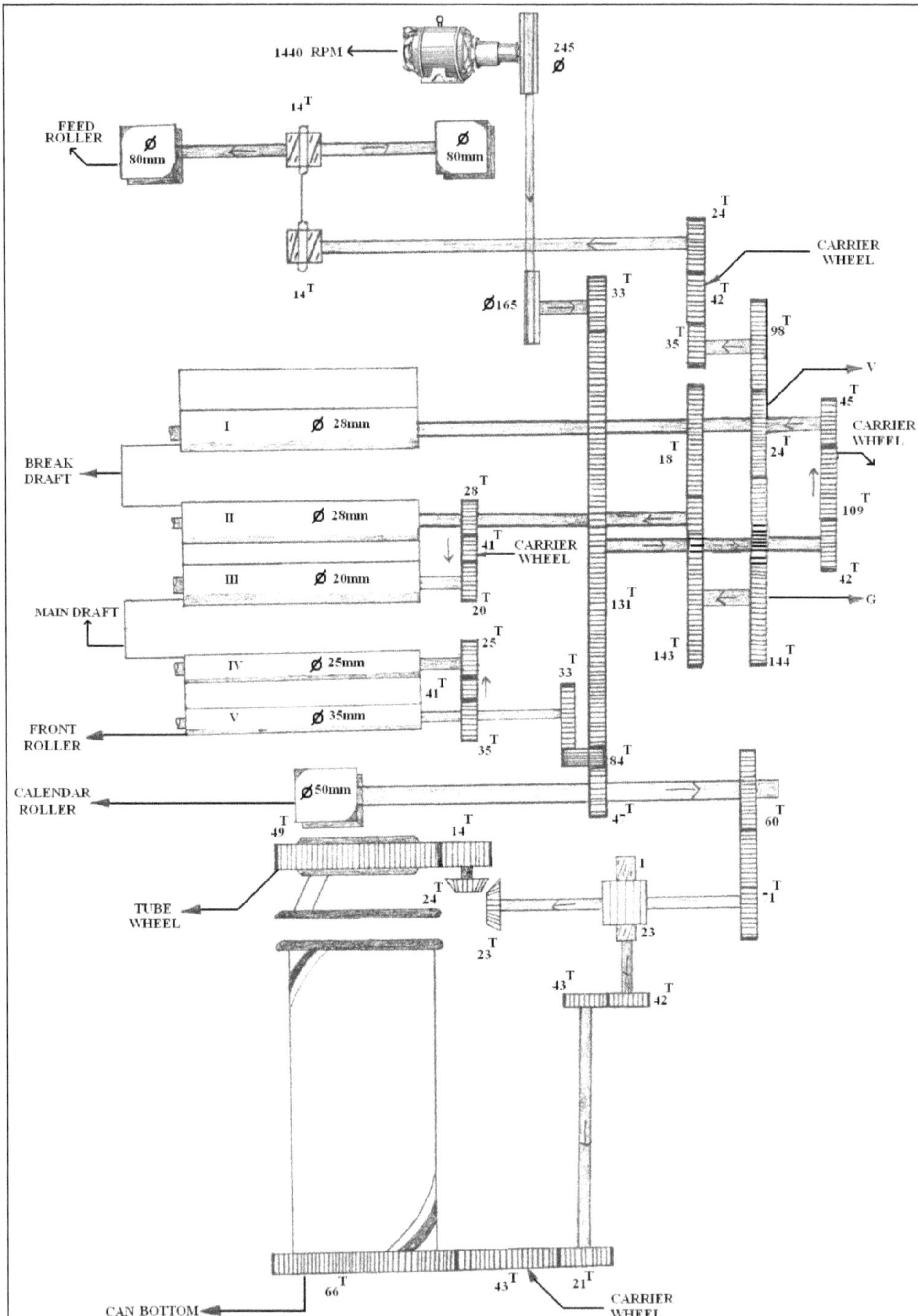

Figure 11.5: High Speed Draw Frame.

12

Study of Roller Setting in Draw Frame Drafting System

1. AIM

- ☆ To observe the design features and important functional elements of the machine / mechanism.
- ☆ To study the roller settings and its effect on yarn quality in draw frame.
- ☆ To study the roller settings for cotton and blends.

2. FORMULA

Refer spinning useful formula relevant to your experiment

3. DESCRIPTION

Drafting Arrangements

The drafting arrangement is the heart of the drawframe and thus the part which exerts the most decisive influence on quality. The requirements placed on the drafting arrangement in general are correspondingly high:

- ☆ Simple, uncomplicated construction;
- ☆ Stable design with smooth running of the rollers (centricity);
- ☆ A mode of operation producing a high-quality product even at high running speeds;

- ☆ High degree of flexibility, *i.e.* suitability for all raw materials, fiber lengths, sliver hanks, etc., that might be processed in the short staple spinning mill;
- ☆ Optimal control over the movement of the fibers during the drafting operation;
- ☆ High precision of both operation and adjustment;
- ☆ Rapid and simple adjustability of roller spacings and draft levels;
- ☆ Ease of maintenance and cleaning;
- ☆ Optimal ergonomic design.

Roller Setting

Drafting roll distances have to be set as close as practicable to control the short and floating fibres, Not so close as to break the longest fibres, nor Not so close as create high drafting forces and over control.

The roll setting has to be optimized according to:

- ☆ Staple length, (2.5% on HVI or AFIS and 1.0% on the Peyer AL-101)
- ☆ Fibre orientation,
- ☆ Sliver weight
- ☆ Fibre crimp, bulk and cohesion.

The number of fibre hooks are decreased and the degree of fibre orientation is increased each drawing process. Therefore, it is necessary to set the roll spacing with this in mind.

Setting Tip

From the practical setting perspective, the main draft rolls should be set first, followed by the setting of the break draft zone. Any change of the distance between rolls (5) and (6) automatically changes the distances between rolls (4) and (5). Consequently, a change of setting of the main draft zone must be followed by an adjustment of the break draft rolls. The converse is not so. A change of the distance of the break draft zone does not change the positions of rolls (5) and (6).

The Main Draft Zone Roll – Setting (H V D)

- ☆ The main draft rolls have an actual minimum setting of 35.5 mm, which is used for all fibres with staple length shorter than 27 mm.
- ☆ For fibres of staple length 27 mm or longer, the rolls are normally set at 8 ....10 mm over the 2.5% length value.

Break Draft Zone - Roll Setting (V V D)

- ☆ The break draft roll setting is dependent upon the condition of the supplied sliver. The maximum and average staple lengths, the degree of fibre orientation, the fibre hooks, the drafting resistance, and the draft distribution all have an influence on how close the rolls can be set. A simple test for the break draft resistance is to use a 1 or 2 mm feeler gauge and push it between the first and second rolls into the slivers. The fibres should yield but with

Roll settings and draft recommendations

Material	Max. staple length mm	Process drawing	Doubling	Feed ktex	Total draft V	Break draft VV	Main draft roll setting HVD	Break draft roll setting VVD
100% comber noil	23	I RSB	4	6	4,9	1.28	35,5	37
Intimate blend 65% CO / 35% comber noil CO waste	38	I SB	4-6	4,5 - 6	4-6	1.16	37	37-38
		II RSB-D 30	4-6	4,5-6	4-6	1,16 (1,057)	37	37-38
CO carded, with high amount of short fibres	34	I SB	6	5	5-5,5	1,28	37,5	39
		II RSB-D 30	6	5	5-5,5	1,16	37,5	42
Peru Tanguis carded (_)= 8 doubling	spin-staple approx. 34...39	I SB	6-8	4,3	6-8	1,28 1,16	38	43 47
		II RSB-D 30	6 (8)	4,3	6 (8)	(1,28)	38	(44)
CO Combed 1 1/16"	36	I RSB-D 30	6	4,2	7,1	1,16	38	45
Egyptian CO, combed SL 2,5% = 34,6 mm SL 50% = 18,5 mm	38-39	I RSB-D 30	8	5,3	8	1,16	40	52
	43	I RSB-D 30	8	4,2	8,3	1,16	44	52
50% cotton combed 50% PES 1,7 dtex/ 40 mm	38/39	I/II SB	8	5	8	1,41 /1,28	43	48
		III RSB-D 30	8	5	8	1,28-1,41	44	50
50% cotton 1 1/16"carded 50% modal 1,3 dtex/ 38 mm	38	I/II SB	8	4	8	1,41	42	46
		III RSB-D 30	8	4	8	1,28	41	48
CV (viscose) 1,3/40 mm	38	I SB	8	4,9	9	1,41	43	46
		II RSB-D 30	8	4,7	8,3	1,28	44	48
PAC 1,3 dtex/ 40 mm crimped	38	I SB	6	4,6	6,8	1,70	44	48
		II RSB-D 30	6	4	6,7	1,28	44	50
PES 1,9 dtex/ 38 mm crimped	38	I SB	8	4,8	8,4	1,41	43	50
		II RSB-D 30	8	4,6	8	1,28	43	50
Sewing thread PES 1,3 dtex/ 38 mm	38	I SB	6	3,8	6,4	1,70	44	50
		II RSB-D 30	6	3,6	6,4	1,70	44	48
PAC 3,3 dtex/ 60 mm, crimped, dyed	spin staple approx. 53/54	I SB	6	5,0	6	1,70	58	65
		II RSB-D 30	6	5,0	8	1,41	58	65

Minimum setting values in mm

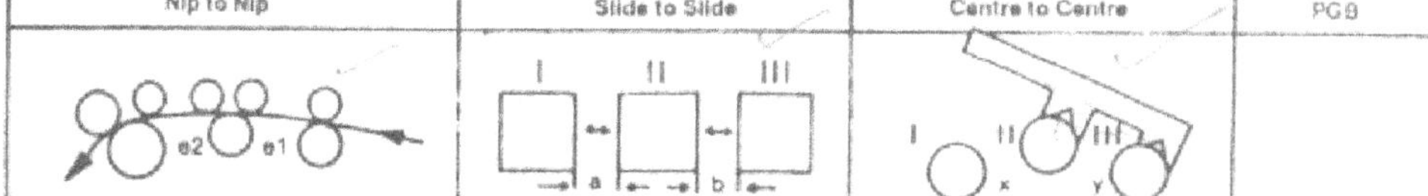

Nip to Nip		Slide to Slide		Centre to Centre		PGB
FRONT ZONE e2	BACK ZONE e1	FRONT ZONE a	BACK ZONE b	FRONT ZONE x	BACK ZONE y	h
38	35	10	3	51	46	0-1,5

Figure 12.1: Recommended Roller Settings and Draft in Draw Frame.

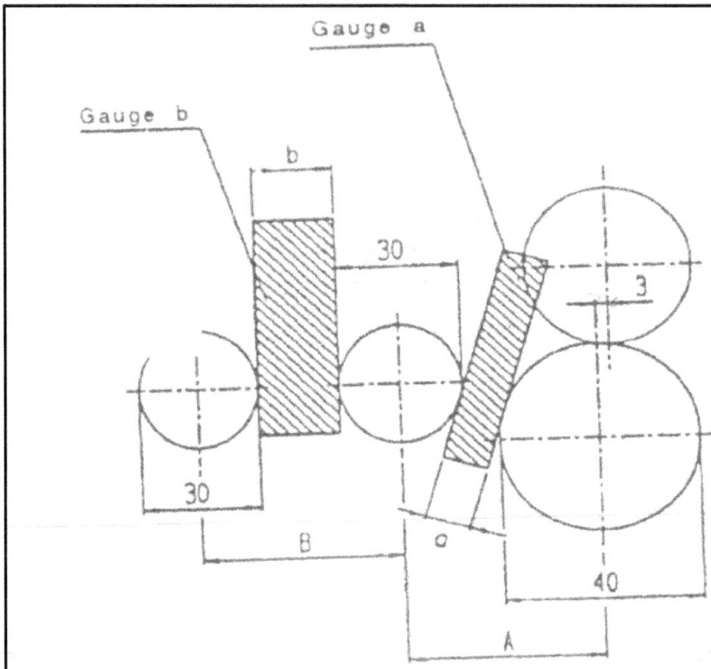

Main Draft		Preliminary Draft	
Gauge	Distance	Gauge	Distance
a	A	b	B
2.5	36	10	40
3.5	37	12	42
4.5	38	14	44
5.5	39	16	46
6.5	40	18	48
7.5	41	20	50
8.5	42	22	52
9.5	43	24	54
10.5	44	26	56
11.5	45	28	58
12.5	46	30	60
13.5	47	32	62
14.5	48	34	64
15.5	49	36	66
16.5	50	38	68
17.5	51	40	70
18.5	52	42	72
19.5	53	44	74
20.5	54	46	76
21.5	55	48	78
22.5	56	50	80
23.5	57	52	82
24.5	58	54	84
25.5	59	56	86
26.5	60	58	88

Figure 12.2: Roller Setting.

resistance. The rolls are too close if the slivers do not allow the feeler to be pressed through.

☆ Closest roll setting is 36 mm

☆ Common roll settings range from 10...15 mm over the 2.5% staple length.

Roller Pressure

The top rolls are pressure - loaded against the bottom rolls to grip the fibres between the rolls and to increase the fibre bundle pressure in the drafting zone. The pressure should not be excessive, but has to be sufficient to maintain a consistent drafting action.

The following points should be noted:

☆ Rolls 1, 2, and 3 are pre set to 320 N,

☆ Deflection roll 7 is preset to 200 N,

For conditions of high drafting forces, such as, low draft ranges, heavy sliver weights or fibres that have a strong drafting resistance the top roll pressure has to be increased to:

☆ Top rolls 1 and 2 to 440 N,

☆ Top roll 3 to 320 N,

☆ Deflection roll 7 remains at 200N.

When the top roll pressure is increased the effective nip zone is extended reducing the distances between the nip points. To compensate for this, it may be necessary to increase the draft roll settings by 1 or 2 mm.

Increasing the roll pressure increases the temperature or the rolls, Lifetime of top rolls is reduced, Top roll deformation will occur if roll pressure is left on when the

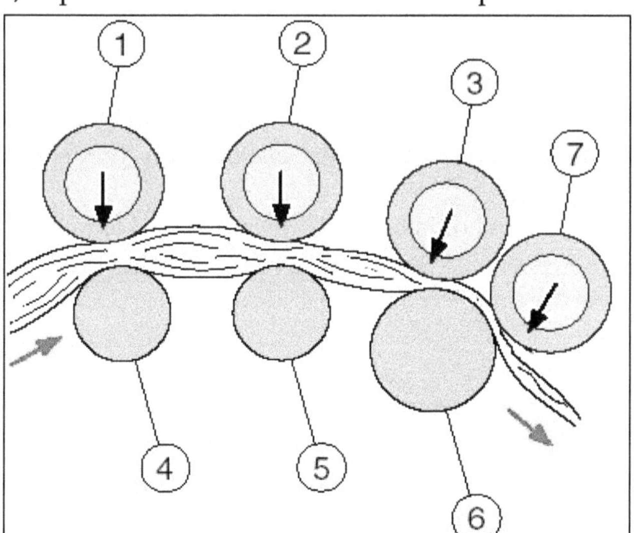

Figure 12.3: Draw Farme Drafting System.

machine stops. With the pneumatic top roll loading system, the pressure is automatically released. This prevents the formation of flat spots on the cots.

Speed

Speeds of the Drawframe have been progressively increased. In most cases the maximum speed of the Drawframe is limited by:

- ☆ The running condition, which is fibre dependent, or
- ☆ The sliver quality that can deteriorate as the speed exceeds optimal levels.
- ☆ Normally, the Draw frames are run at speeds below the maximum rate because the cost of drawing is a relatively small component of the overall spinning costs.

Effects of Excessive Speed

- ☆ Increased top roll laps,
- ☆ Roll temperatures exceed the tolerance of some man made fibres,
- ☆ Increased machine stops and reduced efficiency,
- ☆ Deterioration in sliver quality,
- ☆ Reduced lifetime of the cots,
- ☆ Overheating of the bearings,
- ☆ Guide to maximum Drawframe speeds.

Cot Condition

Top roll cot condition is very important in obtaining an efficient performance of a Drawframe and maintaining an acceptable quality level. The followings should be observed:

- ☆ Top roll cots are selected to produce good quality sliver and to minimize roll laps.
- ☆ Cots can be provided with spiral grooves to reduce the tendency to wrap.
- ☆ a chemical treatment is recommended to smooth the surface.
- ☆ The minimum diameter of the top rolls is 36 mm. They should not be buffed below this limit.
- ☆ Top roll clearers should be used only if required to reduce top roll laps.
- ☆ Clearers increase the temperature of the drafting system and reduce the lifetime of the cots.

4. PROCEDURE

1. Sketch the drafting arrangement of draw frame machine.
2. Mention the setting points in the drafting arrangement.
3. Measure the roller setting in different zones in drafting system.
4. Measure the top roller pressure using the instrument.

5. RESULTS

Tabulate the results.

Zone	*Recommendation of setting*	*Measured setting*
Break Draft Zone		
Main Draft Zone		

Zone	*Recommended pressure (kgs)*	*Measured pressure (kgs)*
Back roller		
Middle roller		
Front roller		

References

1. Werner Klein (2011). *Rieter Manual of Spinning.*
2. Carl A. Lawrence (2003). *Fundamentals of spun yarn technology,* CRC Press, New York.
3. Peter R. Lord (2003). *Handbook of Yarn Production - Technology, Science and Economics,* Textile Institute, UK.
4. T.V.Ratnam (2010). *Norms for spinning mills,* SITRA Publication.
5. Quality management in textile laboratory, Application report, Uster Technologies.
6. Ratnam, T.V and Chellamani, K.P (1999). *Quality control in spinning,* SITRA Publication.
7. T.K. Pattabhiram and T.P.Saiprabha. *Essential Calculations of practical cotton spinning,* Mahajan Publishers Private Limited, India.
8. Operation manual, Rieter spinning system.
9. Rieter Technology Handbook, 2006
10. Operation manual, LMW.
11. www.rieter.com
12. www.lakshmimach.com
13. www.truetzschler.in

www.ingramcontent.com/pod-product-compliance
Ingram Content Group UK Ltd.
Pitfield, Milton Keynes, MK11 3LW, UK
UKHW020821290926
15470UKWH00003B/1299

9 789351 309574